7 Steps to Wellness

Howard J. Rankin Ph.D

**With recipes and nutritional analysis by
Colleen Wracker R.D.**

StepWise Press

Published by StepWise Press
PO Box 4797
Hilton Head Island, South Carolina
SC 29938-4797

(803) 842 7797

First printing, February , 1998

Copyright © 1998 Howard J. Rankin
All rights reserved

Library of Congress Catalog Card Number 97-81418
ISBN: 0-9658261-1-2

Printed in the United States

Cover design by ag2, Hilton Head Island, South Carolina

The author gratefully acknowledges the publishers' permission to quote from the following books.

"Dave Barry's Complete Guide to Guys" by Dave Barry. Random House New York, 1995
"The Road Less Traveled," by Scott Peck M.D. Simon & Schuster, New York, 1978.

Contents

Acknowledgements

I hope this book will meet all your expectations and help you to a healthier, happier life. This psychological and behavioral program is designed to help you stay motivated and to give you all the tools you need to achieve your goals and dreams.

I am a clinical psychologist with more than twenty years experience in helping people change their lives for the better. My experience lies specifically in treating addictions, eating disorders, stress and in mind-body healing. Along the way I have acquired much information on nutrition, exercise physiology and medicine. I am, however, not a qualified professional in these areas. For this reason I have relied on the help of a team of experts in these areas who have guided, verified, and, where necessary, corrected my positions. I am grateful to Roger Sargent Ph.D, and Larry Durstine Ph.D., University of South Carolina, Dr Kent England, Hilton Head Island, Rita DiGiacchino Ph.D., Armstrong Atlantic University, Savannah and Colleen Wracker R.D., who devised the menu plan and recipes.

In addition to these professional colleagues and the many clients who have taught me so much about human nature, I am also indebted to my family who willingly sacrificed time in loving support of my endeavors. So a big thank you to M.J., James, Josh and Ellen without whom this would not have been possible or meaningful.

Introduction

The 7 Steps to Wellness program contains the following elements:

- A detailed description and analysis of the key components to wellness and weight management. These seven steps are; Motivation, Self Management, Self Control, Craving Control, Mindfulness, Binge Management and Dealing with Others

- A set of retraining exercises designed to give you the skills you need to achieve wellness, lose weight and keep it off.

- A complete 14 day menu plan with nutritional analysis of each meal, snack suggestions and a composite grocery list.

- A comprehensive plan of detailed physical exercises.

- A guide to sensible exercise, good eating and healthy behaviors.

- A Personal HealthScope that helps you keep track of your health goals on a daily basis.

- A Dining Out guide that provides general tips for eating out as well as specific guides for the popular ethnic restaurants.

Other considerations

The nutrition plan developed by dietitian Colleen Wracker is an excellent, low-fat healthy menu. *If however, you have special food needs, for example, allergies or medical conditions that require particular dietary considerations, consult your physician or dietitian before following our menu plan.*

The exercise plan included in this program includes some simple stretching, some resistance exercises and walking. *You should consult your physician before starting any exercise program. Follow the program guidelines to ensure that you work at an appropriate level of exertion and without discomfort.*

The mental retraining exercises involve certain assignments. *Only do these assignments if you feel comfortable doing them.*

The program will get you thinking about your thoughts, attitudes and behavior. The program will provide some answers and guidelines for managing change but you may have particular issues and concerns that can not be addressed by a program of this nature. *In the event that you are concerned about some of these issues, you are encouraged to seek the advice of a qualified, licensed psychologist or other mental health practitioner with an expertise in the treatment of weight and eating disorders.*

Using this book as a fourteen day program.

The book is structured in such a way so that you can use it as a fourteen day program. Use the Personal Healthscope's fourteen days to structure your program. Complete the Healthscope each day and then follow the schedule listed below. You can strictly follow the fourteen day menu plan or use it as a guide

Day 1: Read pages 8-18 and 147-186. Do aerobic assessment test on page 173.

Day 2: Read Motivation chapter and do the exercises. Walk. Do muscular endurance assessment (p. 179).

Day 3: Read Self-Manangement chapter and do the exercises. Do the resistance exercise routine starting on page 179.

Day 4: Read the Mindfulness chapter and do the exercises. Walk. Do the flexibility routine starting on page 177.

Day 5: Read the Binge Management chapter and do the exercises. Do the resistance exercise routine. Walk

Day 6: Do the flexibility exercises. Review motivation exercises. Walk

Day 7: Review your week as outlined in the Personal Healthscope. Review the self-management exercises starting on page 49. Do the resistance routine.

Day 8: Read the Self-Control chapter and do the exercises. Walk

Day 9: Review Binge Management exercises starting on page 86. Walk. Do the flexibility routine.

Day 10: Read the Coping chapter and do the exercises. Walk.

Day 11: Read the chapter on Dealing with Others, do the exercises. Do resistance exercises.

Day 12: Walk. Do the Flexibility routine. Read the chapter on Wellness for the Family.

Day 13: Review self-control (p.108) and coping exercises (p. 127). Walk. Resistance exercises.

Day 14: Review your week as outlined in the Personal Healthscope. Review the self-management exercises. Do the resistance routine. Congratulate yourself!

Completing the program once will give you a great start on your weight mangement efforts but you will need to continue the physical and mental exercises to really establish your new behaviors.

What is Wellness?

Wellness is a state of mind. It is a commitment to make healthy choices a priority in your daily lifestyle decisions. Wellness involves taking preventive measures rather than waiting until you are sick to consider your health. Wellness is incorporating into your life those behaviors that have been shown to benefit your mind and body and eliminating those actions known to have a detrimental effect. In short, wellness is nothing more or less, than committing to make your body and your mind the best it can be.

The basics of a good wellness regime are outlined in the program guide but to quickly review them here, they include:

⇒ Eating a diet low in fat, particularly saturated fats - getting no more than about 25% of your daily calories from fats, and no more than 10% from saturated fats.

⇒ Eating five fruits and vegetables a day or at least supplementing your diet with antioxidants, vitamins C and E and Beta Carotene. These practices seem to have cancer prevention characteristics.

⇒ Minimizing sugar and caffeine in your diet. These deplete you of energy if you take them in more than moderate doses. Energy is critical for your psychological and emotional well-being.

⇒ Exercising "aerobically" for at least thirty minutes a day for a minimum of three days a week. Walking, bicycling and jogging are the most common examples of this type of exercise. There are numerous advantages to exercise, including substantial disease and mortality risk reduction, weight management, and increased energy. Exercise is also the best stress manager

⇒ Doing resistance and flexibility exercises three times a week to preserve muscle, keep supple and prevent muscular and joint related diseases.

⇒ Taking a fifteen minute minimum relaxation break at some point in the workday. This helps you recharge your batteries and provides some stress inoculation and increased energy

⇒ Managing stress and emotions through a range of psychological and physical techniques

⇒ Ensuring that you get an appropriate amount of sleep and rest

⇒ Ensuring that you get the appropriate medical screenings and tests.

Now, none of these behaviors are difficult to do. They are not dangerous, threatening or require any special skills. Yet, many people have the most enormous difficulty incorporating them into their lifestyle. The real key to success is learning how to turn your good intentions into good habits that will last and truly make a difference to the quality of your life.

How to Turn Good Intentions into Good Habits

Everyone wants to get the most out of their lives. Everyone wants to live life to the fullest, to preserve their health and be the best they can be. Everyone wants to look great and feel even better. Most people, however, do not lead a lifestyle that is consistent with these desires.

It is not that we do not know what has to be done for weight control and wellness. We now have a solid body of evidence that tells us exactly what we need to do to be at our best. Facts are not the problem here. The problem is how do you adapt these facts into your lifestyle and apply known wellness principles?

As a clinical psychologist who has helped many people change over the course of my twenty plus year career, I understand the problems people have with change. They know what to do -- it's doing it that's the hard part.

I have discovered that the secret to change is surprisingly simple. The process of change must be made as easy as possible -- the easier it is, the more likely change is.

Change is not about facts, it is about making the development of new behaviors as easy as possible.

This wellness and weight control system was devised with the specific intention of making it as easy as possible for you to develop the right health habits.

I have worked in universities and hospitals and in several academic settings. I know how academics think. They want facts, details and logic and they often devise their programs accordingly. The average person, however, does not always operate logically and is not interested in academic discussion. They just want to be shown how to do it and be given incentives for change.

Adapting good habits does not require that you become a professor of nutrition or an expert exercise physiologist. In my view, a little knowledge can be a dangerous thing. I have seen many people completely sidetracked from their wellness and weight goals by getting too involved in the complexities of nutrition which were neither necessary nor important to their main purpose.

> *Confucius say, "Look not at what men say, but what they do." Rankin agree, but add, "Look not at what men know, but what they do."*

Balance and The Seven Steps

7 Steps to Wellness is not just a wellness program - it is a set of tools that you can use to maximize your performance. I am convinced, on the basis of my own clinical experience in this area as well as my understanding of the scientific literature, that regardless of which particular diet or exercise regimen or stress management techniques you prefer the key issue is your implemetation - how do you develop the behaviors that you want to achieve?

Success requires three main elements - motivation, organization and skills. The Seven Steps show you how to harness your motivation, develop your organizational resources and learn the skills you need to make wellness and weight loss a reality.

In addition to these seven steps, there is an underlying philosophy that is essential in any endeavor including wellness.

The secret to successful management of your health is -- *balance*.

Unfortunately, we live in a society that assumes that more is always better. As far as health is concerned, more is not always better -- in fact, *more is often worse.* For example, megadosing with certain vitamins has shown to have detrimental effects, as does exercising compulsively. The body, like the rest of nature, is a complex system that needs to stay in harmony. Our immune system is designed to work most efficiently when it is in balance. Too little immune system activity results in vulnerability to opportunistic infections, like tuberculosis and influenza and too much immune system activity leads to autoimmune diseases like multiple sclerosis, lupus and rheumatoid arthritis.

Being in balance, having a life that satisfies your important needs, is an essential part of wellness. When you are out of balance you are in danger of falling over.

Wellness and Successful Weight Management

I have never seen someone successfully implement a wellness program whose weight and eating were out-of control. Diet is probably the biggest component of a wellness program for two reasons. First, eating presents a continual challenge to our wellness intentions. At least three times a day, sometimes more, you are faced with decisions and actions that affect your very well-being. If you cannot control what you eat it is going to be difficult for you to achieve your health goals. Second, obesity is associated with the leading causes of mortality - cardiovascular disease, cancer, hypertension and diabetes. If you are overweight, you are increasing the odds of disease, and that is obviously incompatible with wellness.

How Overweight Are You?

The official criteria for obesity is based on the percentage of body weight that is fat. This figure varies for men and women.

A body fat that is more than **22%** of total weight in men.
A body fat that is greater than **32%** of total weight in women

There are various ways of measuring body fat, some use complicated scientific measurements, some use simple instruments like calipers. The easiest guide is to calculate your Body Mass Index (BMI) a good measure of overweight and health risk.

The formula for calculating your BMI is:

Weight in pounds x 705 divided by height (inches) x height (inches)

For example, if a woman was 5 feet 4 inches and weighed 180 pounds her BMI would be..

$$\frac{180 \times 705}{64 \times 64} = \frac{126,900}{4096} = 30.98$$

Category	BMI
Overweight	26 - 26.99
Obese	27 - 29.99
Severely Obese	30 - 39.99

A BMI in excess of 30 is associated with increased health risks.

The Medical Risks of Excess Weight
The medical risks of excess weight are not only based on how much fat you have, but where it is located. Researchers have found that abdominal fat is associated more with health risks than lower body fat. So your body shape has much to do with how at risk you are.

Fat stored around the waist creates an apple shape. Fat stored around the hips and thighs creates a pear shape. The waist-to hip ratio is a measure of whether you are an apple or pear shape and the degree of associated health risk.

The Waist-to-Hip ratio is simply calculated by..
Measuring your waist in inches and dividing that by your hip measurement in inches.

Your waist is measured by measuring yourself from 1 inch below your navel. Your hips are measured by measuring from around the largest protrusion of your buttocks.

A Waist-to-Hip ratio of 1.0 or more in men and 0.85 or more in women is associated with increased health risks.

This is in addition to any health risks you might have as a result of a high BMI. A BMI over 27 is associated with moderately increased health risk, a BMI of 30 is associated with a highly increased health risk and a BMI over 35 is associated with a very highly increased health risk.

The diseases that are related to obesity are diabetes, hypertension, cardiovascular disease, stroke, gallbladder disease, degenerative arthritis and cancer (especially of breast, womb, colon and prostate).

It is obvious, therefore, that if you are serious about leading a healthy lifestyle you have to reach and maintain a sensible, health weight. (i.e. a BMI between 20 and 27).

Using the following formula you can calculate your ideal BMI range.

Lower range (BMI of 20) = $\dfrac{20 \times \text{your height(in inches)} \times \text{your height}}{705}$

Someone who is 64 inches tall, this would be: $\dfrac{20 \times 64 \times 64}{705}$ = **119**

Upper range (BMI of 27) – $\dfrac{27 \times \text{your height(in inches)} \times \text{your height}}{705}$

Someone who is 64 inches tall this would be: $\dfrac{27 \times 64 \times 64}{705}$ – **156**

The range for a person who is 5 feet 4 inches is therefore, 119 to 156 pounds. The mid point of that range is 137 pounds.

These numbers are intended to give you a guide, especially as to the relationship between weight and health risks. Numbers and goals are one thing, actually putting an effective weight management program into practice is another. So, first, let us consider what it takes to eat a healthy diet and lose excess weight.

> **Balance is the secret to winning the battle of the scales.**

"How much weight do I need to lose?" That's the first question people ask themselves when they are getting ready to tackle a diet. Unfortunately, it is the wrong question. The question should be,

"What level of eating and exercise can I realistically expect to maintain?"

Once you have answered that question you can determine a realistic rate of weight loss and performance. A weight chart may tell you that you are thirty pounds overweight. Your lifestyle may only support a weight loss of three pounds a month, so realistically you need to accept that it is going to take almost year to drop the weight. Of course, most people don't want to accept that. So they say themselves, "I want to lose that thirty pounds in the next month," and try to set up an regimen that will achieve that goal, only to find that the regimen is impossible to maintain for more than a day or two.

The secret to being successful at weight control is to recognize what is possible for you and to set up a program accordingly.

Your rate of weight loss can be determined by considering the following formula:

Caloric intake per day (the food you eat) - Energy expenditure (metabolic rate, the calories your body expends keeping you alive + activity level)

Suppose you eat 1200 calories a day (the more fat in your food the more calories you will consume)

Suppose your metabolic rate is 1000 calories a day. (Most women over 35 have a metabolic rate somewhere between 900 and 1300 calories daily. Men over 35 have a metabolic rate in the range of 1400-1900 calories a day. No, it's not fair is it?)

Suppose you are moderately active, walking two miles, three times a week and are not completely sedentary. You spend another 500 calories a day. On the formula, your rate of weight loss can be calculated as follows:

1200 - 1000+500 = -300. On this regimen, you are burning 300 calories a day more than your eating.

If you did this for seven days, at the end of the week, you would have spent 2100 calories (300 x 7) more than you would have eaten. Because they are 3500 calories in a pound you would have lost 2100/3500 of a pound or 0.6 pounds!

Unfortunately, most people balk at that. They want to lose it quicker. They want to lose thirty pounds in a month. Let's see what they have to do to achieve that.

To lose thirty pounds in a month requires a deficit over that period of 105,000 (30 x 3500) calories or 3500 calories a day. To be in a deficit of 3500 calories a day you could:

Eat 0 calories and count on burning 3500 calories. Even if your metabolic rate was 1000 calories (and metabolic rate slows down if you starve your body, like this) you would still have to walk approximately 25 miles a day. So to lose thirty pounds in a month you could eat nothing and walk a marathon each day for a month!!

Of course, this isn't a healthy regime, so you could decide to eat 1000 calories a day. The only problem is that you now have to walk thirty-five miles a day!!

I hope that you can see that rapid weight loss is more likely to be a myth rather than a reality.

The example, above, where someone is moderately active, eats on average 1200 calories a day and loses a little more than half-a-pound a week is not glamorous but **it is effective**. If someone stayed on that basic regime, sometimes eating a little more, sometimes a little less, they would lose thirty pounds in a year.

So they key to successful weight control is choosing a plan and a lifestyle that is manageable. There is no point in going to extremes to lose weight, because the chances are extremely high that you will put it all back on again after you return to a manageable lifestyle.

The menu plan that we have provided with this program allows for between 1000 and 1400 calories per day. There is some flexibility in there to allow occasional snacks and treats.

With these thoughts in mind, here are my ten weight control recommendations that have been the most helpful to my clients.

1. Be realistic with your weight goals.
You are only likely to be able to maintain the lowest adult weight that you have ever maintained.

2. Lose weight slowly.
I know you want to lose all that excess weight by the end of the week, if not sooner but *the slower you lose the weight, the more likely you are to keep it off.* A good rule of thumb, is expect to lose 1% of body weight per week. For example, if you weigh 200 pounds, a realistic expectation would be a weight loss of 2 pounds per week.

The following factors influence the *speed* at which you will lose weight. *They do not mean that you can not lose weight. Don't use them as an excuse for not trying.*

> Hormonal changes (including menopause)
> Hormone therapy
> Childbirth
> Quitting smoking
> Medications
> Metabolic conditions
> Aging

Following this program will help modify some of the slowing effect of these factors.

3. De-emphasize weight and focus on wellness and well-being.
Even if you do not know it yet, the most important thing is how you feel. Feeling good should be your main goal. Remember, it's the habit that you want -- weight loss will follow the development of the appropriate habits.

4. Weigh no more frequently than once a week.

The scales are an unreliable measure of weight loss, in the short term. *It takes anything from a few hours to a few days, and sometimes even a few weeks, for the scales to register that you have indeed lost fat*[1]. Even though the scales do not show it, you may still have burned excess fat. Don't get hooked on the scales!

5. Just focus on the immediate goal.

Divide your goal into 5 pound segments, and just focus on losing the next five pounds. If you don't think 5 pounds is a lot, carry a five pound bag of sugar (or anything else) around for an hour.

6. Concentrate on behavior not weight.

If you are doing the right things you will reach the right weight for you and feel great.

7. Establish "maintenance"

Do not be on the weight loss phase of this or any program for too long. You need to establish a maintenance pattern, so that you don't regain your weight when you stop being on "on a diet." It is essential to have periods where you are content simply to maintain your weight rather than lose it. In addition, establish a limit over above you will not go. *Drawing the line against "weight creep" is crucial for long-term success and is the way that successful people prevent getting out of control.*

8. Don't be a perfectionist

You are not perfect. There will be times when you do not eat or exercise the way you had   hoped. Do not give up or get discouraged. Success at anything requires perseverance. I have known many people who have lost and maintained a lot of

---

[1]When fat is burned out of a cell it creates a vacuum that is soon filled with water. Because water is heavier than fat, merely weighing, will not tell you that you have burned fat. Eventually, when the water has been passed out of the cell, the cell shrinks and weighing will indeed tell you that you have burned fat/lost weight. It takes anything from a few hours to a few days (sometimes longer) for this process to occur. So, it is possible, even likely, that on some occasions you will burn fat, but this fat loss will not be reflected in the scales.

weight, and everyone of them will tell you that they had times when they were not in control. Rather than get discouraged, these successful folks would simply get back on track as soon as possible.

9. You have the power to change

The *7 Steps To Wellness* program does not require you to do anything beyond your power. In fact, you are probably doing most of these things already -- you are just not doing them consistently enough to make a difference. You can be successful.

10. Use all aspects of this program.

The motivational component is crucial in helping you stay focused on your goals.

The nutrition plan is a sensible, manageable way of controlling your weight and getting healthy.

The exercise recommendations will help you reach your weight goals.

The training exercises will teach you the new behaviors you need.

Step One

Motivation: Finding the Magic

As a clinical psychologist I have worked with hundreds of people in hospitals, in private practice, in wellness retreats and in academic institutions. Wherever I have worked I have found that people want two things. They want to get more control over their lives and they want some sort of magic to help them get it.

Yes, most people want magic. Our world of rapidly developing technology fuels our fantasies that the magic exists -- that the answer to our health and weight can be found in a pill, or a simple book, or a piece of exercise "equipment" that costs $19.95. Unfortunately, that sort of magic does not exist, neither is it ever likely to. But there is a magic -- a magic that works everyday and I've seen it. I've seen it regularly throughout my career as a clinical psychologist helping people with all types of problems from eating disorders to depression and working with people who are just trying to gain some control in their life. The magic is often right there in front us but we are too short-sighted to see it.

So I have been fortunate enough to see the magic at work. How else can you describe what happened to a female client of mine. This was a person who, after struggling with her weight all her life, embarked on a wellness program consisting of sensible eating and exercise, proceeded to lose over a hundred pounds, while changing her life by divorcing her husband and becoming a single working mother with four growing children to care for. Or how about the businessman, an inveterate smoker for forty years, who simply decided to quit and gave up forever with barely a withdrawal symptom?

All of us know people who seem to have been magically transformed and are achieving almost undreamed of success in their attempts to look good and feel even better. The magic for all of these people was not a chemical concoction or a piece of stretchy rubber, although they may have used these as helpful tools. No, the magic was not an external commodity -- the magic was totally and completely, within them.

How to Make Magic

I will tell you right up front that the key to magic is motivation. If you can allow yourself to mine your motivation and unleash it's terrific force, magical things can happen to you.

This section on motivation may just be the most important part of the program. Most people have a good idea what they need to do to lose weight and lead a healthy lifestyle. In fact, you could summarize the recipe for a successful diet in two simple phrases - eat less fat and exercise more. But knowing what to do and actually doing it are two completely different things. The problem that people have with their diets and their attempts to be healthier is, by and large, not a problem of knowledge but a problem of motivation. In this chapter and the accompanying exercises I will help you mine and capture your motivation.

It is very important from the outset that you need to understand some aspects of motivation in general and your motivation in particular. First, you do have motivation. Yes, I know that sometimes it does not feel like you have but you do. You would not be reading this if you did not have some motivation. The secret to being successful is finding the motivation inside you, capturing it and keeping it in the forefront of your mind enough of the time to make a difference. Motivation is not a fixed asset that you either do or do not have. Motivation fluctuates.

Being successful at anything requires a combination of knowledge, motivation and skills. Knowing what to do and having the skills to do them is one thing but if you do not find your motivation, all the knowledge and skills in the world will not help you.

The Basics of a Healthier Life

A healthy lifestyle, simply put, is incorporating into your life those behaviors that have been shown to benefit your mind and body and eliminating those actions known to have a detrimental effect. In short, this is nothing more or less, than committing to make your body and your mind the best it can be.

The basics of a good wellness regime are outlined in the program guide but to quickly review them here, they include:

20

⇒ Eating a diet low in fat, particularly saturated fats - getting no more than about 25% of your daily calories from fats, and no more than 10% from saturated fats.

⇒ Eating five fruits and vegetables a day or at least supplementing your diet with antioxidants, vitamins C and E and Beta Carotene. These practices seem to have cancer prevention characteristics.

⇒ Minimizing sugar and caffeine in your diet. These deplete you of energy if you take them in more than moderate doses. Energy is critical for your psychological and emotional well-being.

⇒ Exercising for at least thirty minutes a day for a minimum of three days a week. This exercise need not be done aerobically but it needs to involve continuous movement. Walking, bicycling and jogging are the most common examples of this type of exercise. There are numerous advantages to exercise, including substantial disease and mortality risk reduction, weight management, and increased energy. Exercise is also the best stress manager.

⇒ Taking a fifteen minute minimum relaxation break at some point in the workday. This helps you recharge your batteries and provides some stress inoculation and increased energy.

→ Ensuring that you get an appropriate amount of sleep and rest.

⇒ Taking appropriate preventive measures and getting timely medical check-ups.

Now, none of these behaviors are difficult to do. They are not dangerous, threatening or require any special skills. Yet, many people have the most enormous difficulty incorporating them into their lifestyle.

Change and Courage
Change is difficult. We get entrenched in our habits and are reluctant to change them. We are also programmed, either by habit or genetics - probably a combination of both, to seek out unhealthy food choices, less active pursuits and more stressful lives.

Much of what we are faced with is the battle between our genetics and short-term gratification on the one hand - and our rationality and long-term planning on the other. Resisting the pull of the short-term often takes courage. It is here that the possibility exists, if you can be really courageous, of finding your magic. It is when we can let our rationality -- the one characteristic that separates us from other animals-- let our rationality control our programmed impulses, that really great things can happen to us. And they can happen to us in any area of our life.

Sometimes we are not able to summon the courage to abandon entrenched positions or even old habits. This was brought home to me some years ago when I met a well-known professional football coach. This man had motivated and cajoled both professional and college athletes to peak levels of performance but when it came to himself - he could not quit smoking. When I asked why he couldn't do this he simply said, "I don't have the courage." He died shortly thereafter of a smoking related illness.

Just because making the change is sometimes difficult is, of course, no reason for abandoning the attempt. Being successful in business, being successful in anything does not come easily -- but that's hardly a satisfactory reason for not trying. Often, when people try to change their wellness habits they experience a natural withdrawal, sometimes physical sometimes psychological, that they mistake for lack of motivation.

For example, just recently I was helping a successful executive to quit a long term sugar habit. She was finding the going rough and on the third day, said, "I do not think I am really motivated. I really would give anything for a sugar fix right now." What she did not realize, until I pointed it out to her, was that this desire for sugar was a perfectly normal and natural phenomena based on her body's expectations of sugar. It had absolutely nothing to do with her motivation. The fact that she had not indulge her sugar craving despite the onslaught from his body was a great testimony to the strength of her motivation! If you like cheesecake and have salivated over the thought of it habitually, this response is not likely to vanish overnight. Neither does it mean, though, that you have no power to change how you react to this response. *Accepting this fact is crucial to effective life management.*

Change is possible. We get caught in thinking habits - of assuming that we always have to think and react as we always have - as if there is some predetermined, immutable path on which we are stuck. Clearly, change is possible. You have changed in many ways over the years. You need to keep in mind the fact that your past responses are your past responses - they do not have to be part of your future.

Recently, a woman who was trying to lose weight said to me; "Dr. Rankin, I just can't see myself as ever being thinner - this is the real me." I told her that overweight image and pattern of response was not the real her - it was simply the *historical one*.

A Five Stage Model of Motivation
In the last fifteen years researchers in the behavioral sciences have developed a simple, five-stage model of motivation for change. The model is appropriate in describing any motivational state and was derived by two researchers Dr. James Prochaska and Dr Carlo DiClemente at the Universities of Texas and Rhode Island. The five stages of motivation are:

1. Pre-contemplation, in which through ignorance or denial there is no desire to even consider change.

2. Contemplation, in which there is consideration of the possibility of change.

3. Preparation, when there is recognition that change needs to occur and preparation for action take place.

4. Action, in which the appropriate action, in this case the development of new behaviors, is taken.

5. Maintenance, where the required action to maintain change is implemented. In many ways maintenance is the hardest phase - it is often less glamorous and exciting and may seem to have fewest initial rewards.

The key question in addressing motivation is what prompts people to move from one stage to the other -- particularly, what prompts them to move from pre-contemplation to contemplation and from contemplation to preparedness and action?

In my opinion, *people change when they experience a conflict in their values, attitudes and behavior.*

Consider this story of a client of mine who told me how she stopped a damaging compulsive eating pattern. This woman was carpooling her seven year-old son and some of his friends and eating candy bars as she was driving. One of her son's friends noticed her eating and somewhat indelicately said, "My mom stopped eating candy bars because she was getting too fat."

At that moment the woman looked down at her son and could see the embarrassment in his eyes. In that moment, what flooded into her consciousness was a strong desire not to embarrass herself, or her son. What flashed through her mind was a determination to change.

Now, she could just as easily have stopped the car, told the tactless child to get out and walk home - but she did not. I do not know why she did not - but, fortunately, she experienced the event in a meaningful way rather than continue with her blind habit.

When faced with such disparity people need to change. The problem is that many of us can distract ourselves from these discrepancies with the business of our lives. Periodically we will be faced with the conflicts. We catch our reflection in the mirror and cringe at what we see. We start feeling the early signs of chest pain, we cough up blood but unless we can capture those conflicts, those critical moments, they will disappear or be pushed back into our subconscious without effecting any drive to change. *The secret to the real magic is, therefore, confronting the conflict of values, capturing the long-term rationality and keeping it in front of us at all times.*

This problem is not confined to wellness. It is about the process of staying focused on what is important to us when they are too many other distractions. It is about the process of staying focused when we are seduced by the allure of short-term gratification.

24

The key to changing your lifestyle successfully is to capture the reasons for your long term goals and motivation, and keep them in front of you at all times.

All this is well and good and somewhat high-minded. In practical terms how do you do this?

Mining Your Motivation

The first rule of staying focused and mining your motivation is to know what your motivation is. Why do you want to control your weight? Do you want to lose weight because you want to minimize your disease risk? Or is it that you want to look better? Perhaps you want to get into smaller clothes size. Perhaps you just want to be around to see your grandchildren grow up. Perhaps you are the sort of person who likes to do the best you can and doesn't like feeling that there is more you could do to improve your life. Reasons are personal. It doesn't matter whether those reasons are health reasons, or vanity reasons, or emotional reasons, they are real motivation.

Once I asked a roomful of participants in one of my programs for their reasons for wanting to lead healthier lives. The first three people responded quite differently.

The first, was a woman in her mid-twenties. She had diabetes and was terrified at the prospect of having to inject herself with insulin. The image of self-injection was her motivation. She just did not want to have to do that.

The second person was a man in his mid-forties. He was fairly active but somewhat overweight and was facing a hip operation if he did not get into better shape. He wanted to avoid the operation as long as possible.

The third person was a man in his sixties who was very overweight. His motivation? To be able to bend down and tie his own shoes.

No doubt everyone else in their room had their own reasons. Note that they all had a reason and it represented a source of discomfort to them. *In fact, the more uncomfortable the reason, the more potential power it has as a motivator.* The problem with uncomfortable thoughts

25

is that we do not like to think about them and we distract ourselves from thinking about them. If we are successful at distracting ourselves from these problems *we will not be in touch with our motivation.*

So the first part of staying motivated and focused is knowing what our motivation is. Having identified that motivation we need to capture it so that it can stay in front of us at all times rather than fade in and out like poor radio reception. If you are like me, when you get poor radio reception, you switch to another station.

One obvious way of keeping this in front of you is by writing it down and keeping it prominently displayed. For example, writing your wellness motivation on the bathroom mirror or displaying it on the refrigerator.

Other ways of keeping these verbal messages in front of you include making a tape to yourself and playing this periodically to remind yourself of your main goals. The motivation exercises that accompany this section of the program will guide you through ways of keeping the motivation in the forefront of your mind.

Another way of staying focused is highlighted in this story told by Charles Schwab, the industrialist not the discount broker. Schwab had just taken over what was to become US steel and called in a business consultant to analyze the operation for possible improvements. The consultant, a man by the name of Lee, could only come up with one suggestion -- one that was ultimately heartily endorsed by Schwab and his executives. His suggestion? At the beginning of each day write at the top of your To Do list your prioritized list of goals. In this way, you start the day reminded of what is really important to you and where you need to spend your energies. This practice works in a business setting and it can work just as well in a personal setting.

Resistance
The flip side of your motivation is your resistance. What reasons do you have for not wanting to get in shape?

Resistance to wellness and weight loss can take several forms, all of which are colored by personal differences. For many people excess weight will enable them to excuse themselves from behaviors or to

26

avoid thoughts that are otherwise painful or frightening. The most common use of weight in this way is to avoid intimacy. Women in particular assume, often wrongly, that an overweight women is a complete turn-off to a man. An intimate relationship requires making yourself vulnerable and many of us are frightened about exposing ourselves in this way. Excess weight, it is assumed will reduce the chances of being put in a position where you have to deal with romantic and intimate interest from another person. As people discover that they continue to get interest, they continue to increase their weight.

Weight is often used as a weapon, as a way of getting back at someone in your life with whom you are angry. I have met countless people who have retaliated against parents who have pressured them about their weight. The fatter these people get, the more distressed they make their parents. The same tactic is used against partners who make the same demands.

Excess weight can give you an excuse not to do all sorts of things, from socialize to exercise. It sounds like a great excuse but it is of course an example of what in AA is called "stinking thinking". Excess weight can also make you feel powerful or protected in some way.

The motivation exercises included with this program will help you reveal to yourself your motivation and resistance. But having knowledge of your motivation is one thing, applying it is another. How can you keep this motivation going enough of the time to make a difference?

More valuable than written messages are images that pack an emotional punch. Imagery can help to maintain motivation.

The Power of Imagery
In my seminars I teach a process call covert sensitization. In this technique powerful personal images are used to keep motivation in the forefront of the participant's mind. For example, the woman who had early onset diabetes and was afraid of injecting herself with insulin was also a fast food freak. I got her to imagine, not the golden arches, but the golden insulin syringe. She practiced the image on a regular basis until, whenever she found herself driving in or through a fast food place, the image of the insulin syringe surfaced in her mind. This did not always

stop her from buying fast food but it made a significant impact on her eating.

Images representing the worst fears are powerful motivators. Many years ago when I was living in London I had to fight the traffic most nights of the week. Very often I would get upset by reckless and thoughtless driving because I am man and thus programmed to get upset at that sort of thing. When I did this, I could feel my blood pressure soaring and my adrenaline pumping. One day, I saw a terrific picture in medical book of a blocked artery. It really made an impression on me. I made a conscious decision to be mindful of that when I drove in the worst of the London traffic. I decided it was not worth it to get so upset by the behavior of other drivers. If I felt my blood pressure rising I just thought of the picture of that blocked artery and you know what -- the traffic did not seem to matter anymore.

I have had people image heart attacks, intensive care units, social embarrassments, lost opportunities, anything that symbolizes their worst fears of not changing their behavior. These are powerful techniques that work.

Conversely, I also get people to imagine their best dreams that occur as a result of being successful. If you think about it, this is how most people motivate themselves. They see the big prize and can project themselves into the future and want to be there.

Motivational messages and images are powerful and necessary for success. The problem is how to keep them in the forefront of your mind? A motivational tape or talk will typically fire you up for a while but a few hours after the talk the impact is completely lost. That is why I have devised the *motivational link method* - a way of keeping all of this good motivational stuff working for you long after you have forgotten who I am.

The Motivational Link Method uses the two key principles of all human learning; association and repetition. I have devised the motivational exercises in this program to utilize these two fundamental principles. Once you have identified your motivation, and your resistance, we will turn these into personalized messages and images. You then need to associate these messages and images not with some

28

relaxing music, as nice as that would be, but to everyday sounds and images. By linking your motivational messages to sensations that surround you every day, there is a much greater chance that you will be reminded of that motivation far more frequently than if those messages are associated with a piece of music you might play once every six months.

The more you can be reminded about your motivation through everyday associations, the more likely you are to be in touch with your motivation and that is key to your success. The Motivational Link Method is the heart and soul of this program and the exercises that follow are designed to help you find your magic and maximize it.

Developing Your Motivation
In the exercises that follow you will use **The Motivational Link Method** to mine your motivation and keep it in front of you.

Creating Powerful Associations

1. Conscious Motivation
The first exercise involves working out what benefits you expect to gain from following this program. *Complete the following by circling the answers that apply to you. Provide any other answers that are relevant to you in the spaces provided at the end.*

The benefits of leading a healthier lifestyle and controlling my weight for me are....

I will feel better about myself

I will look better

I will be more attractive

I will feel in control

I will like myself

I will be happier

I will be able to wear clothes I like

29

I will have more energy

I will be more active

I will live longer

I will be setting a good example to my children

I will be respected by others

I will.......

Therefore, I want to achieve

....

....

....

Now you have worked out what benefits you will gain from following my program you need to *consider what disadvantages or costs there are if you do not do this.*

When people start out to change they are motivated by wanting to avoid unpleasant negative consequences of their current behavior. A big part of your motivation will come from being aware of what it is you want to avoid and having the courage to face it head on. The next exercise will help you define what you want to avoid by changing your current behavior. Let's look at what you don't like about your current lifestyle.

The Case of the Nighttime Binger

Ms. M came to see me almost in despair. She wanted to lose an excess twenty pounds and get fit. She would start each morning with good intentions, make healthy decisions during the day but as nighttime wore on, she found herself less and less in control. Most nights she would find herself eating a lot of high-fat food. Immediately after this, she felt ashamed and disgusted with herself and completely out of control. She was eventually able to mine these horrible feelings, and by keeping them in the forefront of her mind, used her desire to avoid them as motivation.

The Case of the Wistful Grandpa

Mr.R was in a man in his late fifties. He could not get a proper wellness program going even though he had a strong family history of heart disease. He would exercise a few times and then stop for months at a time. He would make some good nutritional choices and then eat high-fat desserts. One day, while watching college football, his only grandson said "Grandpa, will you come and watch me when I play football in college?" When he heard this, Mr.R's only thought was of his own father dropping dead of a heart attack at the age of fifty-eight. Mr. R. had just turned fifty-eight. Would he see his grandson graduate from high school let alone college? Would he see him grow up at all? At that moment he made the commitment to do everything he could to take care of himself and lead a healthier lifestyle.

(Complete the following by circling the answers that apply to you. Provide any other answers that are relevant to you in the spaces provided at the end.)

The disadvantages of being out of shape and overweight are...

I will hate myself

I will feel out of control

I will be depressed

I will feel ashamed

I will feel guilty

I will feel ugly

I won't fit into clothes I like

I will have no energy

I will not have friends

I will get sick

I will die younger

I will get fat

I will be wasting my life

I will be setting a bad example to my children

I will not be respected by others

I will.......

Therefore, I really want to avoid

....

....

Therefore I want to embark on this program because:

I want to achieve

....

....

I want to avoid....

....

....

Well Done! What you have just written is your motivation and it is crucial to your success. It is your *rational anthem* and just like the national anthem, you need to learn it by heart and be moved each time you think about it. Now you have created your first associations, they need to be reinforced with repetition.

Rankin's Repetition Reminder:
Review the hopes and the fears that you have just identified, every night before going to bed and every day first thing in the morning.

> **Reviewing your goal**
> **Is good for the soul**

2. Creating Catchy Phrases.
A key component of my motivational system is creating catchy phrases that stick in your mind and become *habitual thoughts*. These phrases will *lurk in your subconscious and pop into your mind at the appropriate time to influence your behavior.*

Short rhyming phrases are easy to remember and have the power to elicit your motivation if the two are associated and repeated enough of the time.

Below, I have supplied some catchy phrases that cover such aspects of motivation as feelings, appearance, weight, health and self-esteem. If you can create your own, so much the better.

Self-Esteem
Fat on your girth, Depletes your self-worth
An Exercise session, Fights depression
Living Correct, Will earn self-respect

Mood
Eating fat food, Will ruin your mood
You won't be serene, With too much caffeine
Extra dressing, Becomes depressing

Physical appearance
Plenty of fruit Will make you look cute
Improve your appeal, With veggies each meal
Get more active, To be attractive

Clothes

Eat too many fries, You'll be oversize
Not eating light, Makes your clothes tight
 No dessert surprises, Maintains the same sizes

Weight

Lots of batter Will make you fatter
Control your weight, With carbohydrate
Take extra precautions, Eat moderate portions

Health

High fat cheeses, Spread diseases
Arteries go splat! When you fill them with fat
Constant fat snacks, Give heart attacks

Energy

Walk five times a week, To reach your peak
 Energies abound, When you move around
If it's too sweet, It'll make you beat

Exercise

A little hustle, Preserves your muscle
Walk a bit quicker, To train the old ticker
Walk five times a week, To reach your peak

General

It's not hocus-pocus, Just keep your focus
I don't need perfection, To like my reflection
Positive thinking, Keeps me from sinking

Having identified those sayings that work for you, you need to be repeatedly reminded of them. I am now going to get you to take your catchy phrases and place them in strategic places in your life. This will enable you to be exposed repeatedly to these important messages.

Most people respond very well to this exercise. I have known people who have placed these motivational reminders on their bathroom mirrors, refrigerators, even in their cars. One enterprising client even put her reminders on the top of her cookie jar, so that when she found herself looking for cookies she was faced with her motivational reminder, which in her case was:

> **Don't ruin your waist**
> **For a small cookie taste**

(Complete the following by circling the answers that apply to you. Provide any other answers that are relevant to you in the spaces provided at the end.)

I will post my catchy motivational phrases.....

On my organizer

On my bathroom mirror

On my refrigerator

On my dashboard

On my telephone

On my television

On my computer

On my desk/workspace

On my front door

On my checkbook

On my weighing scales

On my kitchen stove

On the back of my hand

On my toothbrush

On the bathroom door

On...

MAGIC TRICK! POST THOSE PHRASES NOW!!

> **The Case of the Supermarket Tape**
> A thirty-year old female client had a lot of difficulty when doing her grocery shopping. Despite her best efforts, whenever she would get into the store she would buy a lot of candy and eat most of it before she even reached the check-out counter. To manage this, she made a tape of her catchy motivational phrases and played them on her headset as she shopped. Result: No more candy.

3. *Creating Powerful Images*

Imagery is a very powerful tool and one that everyone can use to achieve some really amazing results. Did you know that imagery is used by many successful people from all walks of life? Athletes have used it with great success. Research has shown that imagining yourself doing something is very similar to actually doing it. There is evidence that the same nerve pathways are used when you imagine yourself doing something as are actually used in the real life performance of that behavior. Visualization represents the easiest and most powerful rehearsal tool and you can get terrific results using it for just a few minutes a day.

Not everyone imagines or visualizes the same way. So here are some things you need to know about visualizations.

First, some people visualize in black and white and others in color. It does not matter which of these you can do. If you do visualize in black and white, practice may help you switch to color.

Some people visualize in still frame as if they are looking at a photograph, while others see full motion video. Again, it doesn't matter which you start with; practice may help you switch to action video.

Some people's images fill the entire "minds eye" while others only take up part of the visual field. Again, there is no better way. If your images only take up part of the visual field, try moving the image around, making it larger, etc.

Some people can clearly see themselves in their visualizations, as if they are watching themselves in a movie, while others see their images "through their eyes" and don't see themselves from outside of their body. Again, this does not matter but experiment to see what works best for you.

While most people favor visual images some of us are able to conjure up stronger experiences with other senses, like smell or taste. Use whatever works for you. Like anything else, visualization and imagery produce the best results with practice.

We are now going create powerful images that reinforce positive ideas. To do this, we are going create empowering associations with everyday sounds.

Sound	Motivational Message
Shower	Respect your body
Ringing telephone	Feel confident, in demand
Car Ignition	Get going
Flushing toilet	Flush away negative thoughts

When doing these visualization exercises, find a comfortable place where you will not be disturbed[2].

1. **Respect your body.** Imagine that you are getting into the shower. Hear the sound of the water flowing as you turn on the faucet. Feel the water on your body. As the water flows through your hair and down your body appreciate what a marvel of creation the human body is. Appreciate what a wonderful gift it is. As the water caresses your body recognize that you need to *respect your body.*
   Every time you shower remember how important it is to respect your body.

---

[2] The Get Motivated Get Smart Get Slim tape series provides these exercises with the appropriate sound effects.

37

2. **Feel Confident.** Imagine feeling full of energy and vitality. Recall the best you have ever felt. Feel confident. Feel healthy, vital and sexy. Imagine that you are in demand. That people want your company. Imagine how that would feel. Imagine that the phone is ringing with people who want your company.

Every time the phone rings recapture this feeling of confidence

3. **Get Turned On.** Imagine making good food choices. Imagine exercising. See yourself resisting high-fat foods. Imagine getting up at the beginning of each day and making a commitment to be healthy and put the program into practice. Imagine each day getting off on the right foot by eating healthily and exercising. As you make the commitment to take yourself seriously each day you are getting revved up - turning on to the program like turning on your car's ignition.

Every time you start your car recapture this feeling of commitment.

4. **Flushing away toxic thoughts.** Imagine that you are tired and somewhat stressed. It's the end of a long day and you have little energy left. This is the state of mind where you have doubts about your abilities and your chances of success. Negative thoughts begin to enter your mind. But you have the ability to ignore those thoughts. You have the ability to control how you react to destructive thinking habits. Imagine resisting the negative thoughts - pushing them aside. Imagine flushing these toxic ideas down the toilet.

Every time you flush the toilet remember you have the power to control   negative thoughts

Positive Images
You may want to create other positive images that are meaningful to you. I have included a list of images that have been helpful to many of my clients. If these don't apply to you make up your own. Practice often.

Being at your ideal body weight

Being full of energy

Buying smaller size clothes

Being able to walk comfortably

Looking attractive

Making good food choices

Rejecting high fat foods

Staying calm under pressure

Being mentally sharp

Being in control

Feeling good after a workout

Accepting compliments on success

Rankin's Repetition Reminder:
Practice your powerful imagery five minutes in the morning and five minutes just before going to bed.

Illness reversal, With ten minutes rehearsal

Now a short test to see if you have been paying attention.
What are the two great principles that govern human behavior?

What are the five stages of motivational change?[3]

---

[3] *Answers: Association and Repetition: Precontemplation, contemplation, preparation, action, maintenance*

Step Two

Self-Management: Focusing the Lens

If you are going to be successful at any project, you will need to master some important management principles. These principles will help you organize your resources in the most efficient way to get the job done. No doubt, you will have practiced such important management principles as goal-setting, prioritizing, reviewing and project and time management in other areas of your life. But have you considered yourself as the project and applied these same management tenets to help you make your own life more efficient?

This may sound obvious but many people resist the idea of seeing themselves as a project. It is sometimes difficult to objectify aspects of behavior and manage it effectively. This may seem difficult, but unless you are prepared to do it you are not likely to be successful.

There are other barriers to effective self-management techniques. The most important of these surrounds the issue of boundaries.

Developing Appropriate Boundaries

A boundary is a psychological limit. It is where you stop and the rest of the world begins. Your boundaries define you and the limits of your responsibility. If the boundary is too tight and describes a very narrow circle, you are self-centered and narrow in what you are prepared to do for others. If your boundaries are flung far and wide, you take too much responsibility, care too much about what others think and end up sacrificing yourself in the fruitless pursuit of living merely to please others. This is a problem for many women who, as a result, run into difficulties with the management of their life in general and their weight in particular.

Women are raised to be outer directed. Their natural constitution is geared for outer directedness and as a result they are more prone to run into boundary issues - or at least the boundary issue of giving too much of themselves away. This deflects many women from their wellness and weight goals. Their program comes way down on their list of priorities because they themselves are low down on the list of priorities. I once asked a participant in one of my programs where her program fit in her priorities. "I think of my life as a totem pole with my activities ranked in order of priority down the pole. I am not even on the totem pole," she said. Obviously if you are not on the totem pole, you are not going to be successful.

Quite apart from a natural and socially conditioned mindset of personal sacrifice, many women say to me that they feel guilty if they spend time taking care of themselves - that this time should be spent taking care of their family or other people in their life. Well, obviously a regular schedule in which you spend an hour exercising, an hour showering and preparing for the day, an hour at the massage therapist followed by an hour at the beautician followed by an hour with a friend prior to spending an hour in therapy - and all of this while your kids are at home being take care of by a baby-sitter is taking looking after yourself a little too far! But caring for yourself and taking yourself seriously enough to manage your health, both physical and emotional, is what Scott Peck calls smart selfishness.[4]

Not that women are the only ones with boundary problems. The man, being directed to strive in a work setting is likely to give himself up to his work. There is a regular parade through my practice of couples who have lost their way because the husband is overcommitted to work, the mother overcommitted to the children and household tasks, not to mention her job, and they have no time for each other or themselves.

Finding balance in life is difficult. All of us benefit, however, if there is some time in the day just for us - time where we can take care of the necessary maintenance to our mind, body and spirit so that we can be replenished and nourished. When we do this we re-center our relationships in a much better frame of mind. Of course, there will be some days when other activities and events take priority but overall it is crucial that you make time for things that are most important to you.

Poor boundaries are the cornerstone of poor time management, and from the above it should be obvious that time management is an essential part of any project. Poor boundaries lead to over-commitment,

---

[4] The Road Less Traveled by Scott Peck M.D., Simon & Schuster, New York, 1978

over-involvement, poor delegation, poor goal-setting and inadequate prioritizing.

You should not feel guilty for trying to lead a healthy lifestyle. On the contrary, you should feel guilty if you do not make a serious attempt to take care of yourself.. We all have been given a fantastic gift of life and it behooves us to cherish and take care of that gift, to look after our selves and our bodies. If you have a young family, it may seem impossible to you to take an hour a day for yourself - but if you do not look after yourself, your family is eventually going to suffer tremendously.

Smart Selfishness

Guilt feelings create a sense of unworthiness - that not only can you not take the time to look after yourself, you do not deserve to. When your self esteem is low throwing yourself into doing for other people is an easy option. Helping others, particularly if they are appreciative, may give your self-esteem a boost. In my experience, however, such behavior perpetuates poor self-esteem rather than enhances it. Such behavior takes a person who considers themselves an unworthy person and turns them into a person who sees themselves as a helpful, unworthy person.

Consider this story about a middle-aged woman who was the office manager of a large legal practice. Not only did this woman manage the practice but she nurtured many of the paralegals who were under her. This office and the people in it became an increasingly large part of her life. It did not take long before many in the office were seeking her opinion about personal matters as well a business ones. She become a sort of local Dear Abby. This was rewarding at first for the office manager, but it started to overwhelm her. She spent most of the time worrying about the personal lives of her subordinates and of course, she would never say no, if a partner in the law firm asked her to stay late or work at week-ends. She finally started to crack and in my office during a therapy session she sobbed bitterly because she felt everyone was taking advantage of her. "No-one thinks I am important," she cried. "And that includes you," I suggested. With the insight thus made, the woman instantly stopped crying, sat bolt upright in the chair and vowed to take care of her own needs rather than taking care of others exclusively and has not had a problem to this day. Well, this is not Hollywood and I have to admit that was not exactly her reaction - but we had made a start.

Over the course of several months this woman was gradually able to learn that *if she was not going to impose her own limits no-one else was going to do it for her.*

Good self-management, therefore, requires a commitment to a stated goal, adequate planning, prioritizing and ensuring that you have the resources, specifically the time, to get the job done. It is also requires awareness of your own behavior.

Awareness

Much behavior, especially eating behavior, is automatic. The behavior is so habitual that it has almost become involuntary. Moreover, eating often takes place in conjunction with other activities, like watching television or talking, so that you can be easily distracted from what you are putting in your mouth. In the section on bingeing, I describe this in more detail, but for now I want to point out to you how easy it is to distract yourself from really paying attention to what you are doing - especially if you are doing something that is inconsistent with a stated goal.

In a study looking at factors related to relapse conducted some years ago, awareness was shown to be important. The technical term used was "cognitive vigilance" (scientists like to use complex language to describe everyday phenomena.) This study showed that the more vigilant people were about their environment and their behavior the more successful they were likely to be in making lifestyle changes.

Keeping vigilant is crucial for successful weight management. There is a natural human tendency to habituate or get used to doing something - even if you are successful. After a while boredom sets in and you lose your vigilance. This happens constantly on diets. You might start off well, sticking to your program admirably for a few days, or even a few weeks, but before long your interest wanes, you stop being vigilant about your eating and exercise habits and the program begins to unravel. This may happen slowly at first, an extra snack sneaks in, then some desserts, then you are putting butter on your bread and now you're back to 2% fat milk and before you look round you have got completely away from your successful behaviors.

Part of the way to prevent this drift back to old habits lies in motivational techniques described elsewhere in this program. Part of the answer is not embarking on crash diets or radical programs that simply are not possible to implement for more than a few days. Part of the answer also lies in keeping yourself vigilant.

Wellness and weight management programs typically provide a daily log or journal in which to record eating and exercise behavior. Such self-monitoring is generally promoted as a key habit to develop. The evidence suggests that people who self-monitor are more likely to be successful. I recently conducted some of my own research on the relationship between success and self-monitoring. In my years in this business I have found that people self-monitored when they were doing well. When they got off track they only monitored their desired behavior and neglected to record the not such good actions, or else they stopped monitoring altogether. Perhaps self-monitoring is effective only because the *successful* people keep doing it. Or maybe, people who self-monitor are somewhat compulsive in what they do and they are the ones likely to be successful. My research into this matter revealed something fairly obvious. People who self-monitored and *had to show their daily monitoring to some authority* do better than those people whose monitoring is not accountable to anyone. Again, this makes perfect sense - if you are having a bad day and no-one is going to ask to see your journal why bother to write down your difficulties?

Awareness of your behavior is crucial, and keeping a record of it is the best way of staying aware. *Going public is the best way of making sure that you keep your record straight.* This is why doing a program like this with a friend or a group can be so helpful.

Vigilance and awareness are important for other reasons, too. Despite the fact that many people know what a sensible diet is, they do not realize how poor they are at putting this into practice. Some years ago I conducted a study in which women were asked to rate the taste and desirability of different foods arranged in small bowls in front of them. They were left alone with the food in the experimental room and told that, in order to rate the foods, they could eat as much of the food as they wished. The foods were cereal, cheese, chocolate, peanuts, raisins and potato chips. At the end of the session, each subject was also asked to rate how many calories of each food they had eaten. Once the subjects left, the foods were weighed to determine how much of each food had indeed been consumed. Nearly all subjects consistently and significantly underestimated the number of calories of each food that they had eaten, despite the fact they all could accurately report how many calories an ounce of each food contained. In short, they knew the caloric value of foods but could not translate this into realistic information about their own behavior.

Several years ago, more sophisticated studies using technological advances that allow for the accurate measurement of calorie consumption in the past twenty-four hours, confirmed my findings. These studies showed that normal weight individuals systematically under reported their calorie consumption by about 50% whereas overweight individuals underreported their calorie consumption by nearly 100%.

Knowing the calorie and nutritional values of foods and *recognizing portion size*, is a necessary weight management skill.

Goal Setting
Realistic goal setting is a critical part of any project. Many people have unrealistic goals when it come to the rate of weight loss and target weight. The general public have, however, become more realistic about such goals over the last several years. There was a time when most people coming to my seminars wanted to lose all their weight tomorrow. They were disappointed if they could not lose five to ten pounds a week. Now, people recognize the research that shows that weight lost more gradually is going to stay off. Rapid weight loss is not an effective way of making long-term changes.

A weight loss of about one pound a week is realistic. Sometimes you will lose more, sometimes a little less. You will see in the footnote on page 17 that even if you burn fat, this does not immediately show up on the scales. There is a time lag between actually burning the fact and the fat cell shrinking .

Goal setting is the backbone of planning. You need to have a goal for every behavior that you plan to change - exercise, eating, stress management. Goals should be expressed in the form of behaviors (e.g. work-out three times a week) Goals should be short-term, actions to be
45

taken this week. Goals should be specific and written (use the personal healthscope provided in the appendix.) It is important that you set aside specific appointments with yourself, especially for exercise. If you do not make such appointments, exercise time will be pre-empted. Consider these appointments with yourself just as important as those with others. Do not break these appointments unless absolutely necessary. In the exercises that follow you will be encouraged to think of ways to make sure you carry through on your goals. Minimize the possibility of distractions by making it clear to others in your life that this is important time for you that cannot be interrupted.

Some people resist setting goals because they don't like being tied down. A goal is a commitment but not an unchangeable one. You do not have to be inflexible. Think of a goal as a guidance mechanism in a rocket - it launches you on a particular course. That does not mean, however, that course alterations and corrections can not be made in flight.

Review Your Progress

Reviewing the previous week's progress is important. Did you meet the goals you set for yourself in the previous week? Did you exercise the number of times you planned? Did you handle those special situations satisfactorily?

If you did meet your behavioral goals you earn a reward. It is important these rewards be based on meeting short-term goals. Rewards that are based on long term performance, lose their power to influence you. It is not helpful to say to yourself, that you will reward yourself once you have reached your target weight. First, that might be so far in the future that the reward is not effective. Secondly, rewards should be based on your behavior, not on weight loss. If you are doing the right things, everything else, including your weight loss will follow.

Rewards

People have uncommon difficulty with rewards. There are some people who simply cannot give themselves credit for their achievements. For some people, the very act of reaching a goal devalues it. Such a self-effacing position is reminiscent of the Groucho Marx line - "I wouldn't want to join a club that would accept me as a member." Recognizing your efforts and giving yourself a pat on the back is important.

46

There is another group of people who, conversely, celebrate their success with an excess of self-indulgence. These are people who want to go on a world cruise to celebrate the fact that they have just lost five pounds.

Here are some simple rules about rewards. Food is not an appropriate reward. Although it is possible to make food and eating a reward, for example dinner at your favorite healthy restaurant, food and rewards need to be disassociated. Using food as a reward is often a precursor to poor eating and weight gain. You don't want to resurrect that pattern of behavior.

Small indulgences make appropriate rewards. A book, or some music, a massage or a trip to the beauty parlor. *The reward is meant to be a small token of self-acceptance and recognition not a way of accumulating wealth.* The exercises that accompany this program guide you through the process of setting up your self-management meeting including your rewards.

An important part of your weekly meeting is anticipating high risk situations and working out how to cope with them. Travel, house guests, special events can present special challenges to your program. Forethought about how to tackle such situations can make a huge difference. Franklin D. Roosevelt's comment is appropriate in this context: "Perfect planning prevents poor performance." The more you can anticipate and plan, the more successful you will be. This is no different from anything else in your life - the more prepared and well-trained you are, the more likely you are to succeed.

Such planning also includes food planning. One goal on a weight management program, especially the weight loss phase, is to spend as little time as possible, thinking about, deciding about, and being around food. One of the reasons why people do well when they are on diet supplements *during the weight loss phase* is that they do not have to think about food. Once the supplements are stopped, however, weight is regained because the essentials facets of lifestyle change have not been learned.

This book contains a 14 day menu plan. If you are using your own meals, plan them in advance. Planning meals is important fro several reasons. First, it reduces the anxiety of thinking about food when you are hungry and tired. Second, you spend less time thinking about food. The evidence suggests that people who follow a menu plan do better than those who do not. Those on a menu plan do not have to spend time thinking and deciding about food.

Plan as many of your upcoming meals as possible. This will also enable you to make a grocery shopping list. It might also enable you to prepare foods for the week at one cooking session thus minimizing the time spent in contact with food.

A weekly review can take as little fifteen minutes. Making the time to monitor and plan is a reflection of your commitment to take your program and yourself seriously.

The self-management principles described here and outlined in the exercises that follow, may not be very glamorous or exciting but they are necessary.

Becoming a Better Self-Mananger

Maintaining focus is one of the biggest challenges of a behavior change program. In this module, exercises and tasks will be presented that will help you stay focused on your mission to lead a healthier life. The principles of self-management that are covered in this module are universally applicable so you may end up improving more than just your health.

Maintaining focus means a number of things. It means keeping your eye on what you are doing. It means acquiring a sharper image of what you want to achieve. Taking a good picture requires knowledge of the subject you want to capture.

Life is like using a camera: Seek the light, keep steady and stay focused.

Goals

Goals are like guidance mechanisms - they set you out on a particular course and they guide you towards a target. **Remember, however, that the guidance mechanism can always be reset if the original target is compromised in some way.** Goals will keep you on course but they don't have to be maintained if they are going to be damaging to you.

Goals always need to be written and stated in specific behavioral terms.

Example of a well stated goal: "I want to be able to get into a size 10 dress by Christmas."
Example of a poorly stated goal: "I want to get into smaller clothing."

Example of a well-stated goal: "I plan to walk three times a week for thirty minutes a day."
Example of poorly stated goal: "I am going to start walking more."

Which of these is the best way to express the same goal?

1a). I am going to eat fewer fat grams
1b). I am going to eat no more than 40 grams of fat per day

2a). I am going to do ten minutes of toning/conditioning exercises, three times next week
2b). I am going to start to tone up.[5]

In this section we are just going to focus on your goals for the **next seven days**. A big picture is made up of a lot of little dots. If you don't take care of the little dots, the big picture will fade from view.

Write down your goals for the next seven days in the following categories. You can write as many goals as you want in each section, as long as they are specific and manageable.

---

[5] answers; 1b, 2a

Eating

It will be useful to set specific goals for calories and fat grams

(*Examples:*
In the next seven days I am going to:

Follow the menu plan provided with this program
Eat no more than forty fat grams per day
Alternate between thirteen hundred and eleven hundred calories per day.)

Now it's your turn.

In the next seven days I am going to:

1....

....

....

2....

....

....

3....

....

....

4....

....

....

5....

....

....

Exercise

(Examples:
In the next seven days I am going to:

Walk five times for thirty minutes
Spend fifteen minutes doing the weights routine every other day
Take an aqua aerobics class on Wednesday and Friday).

Now it's your turn.

In the next seven days I am going to:

1..
....
2..
....
3..
....
4..
....
5..
....

The Self-Care Lens

Write down all of the other self-care behaviors that you intend to perform in the next seven days.

(Example:
In the next seven days I am going to:

Have one massage
Take one relaxing bath
Read the 7 Steps To Wellness manual for ten minutes each night)

Now it's your turn
In the next seven days I am going to:

1..
....
2..
....
3..
....
4..
....
5..
....

Now that you have your goals for the next seven days, write down on a piece of paper, **exactly when you are going to do each of the behaviors you have listed above.**

The entries you have just written are commitments to yourself. Commitments to yourself are more important than your commitments to anyone else because you only have to spend a few minutes of your time with "them", but you will be living with yourself for the rest of your life. **So the appointments with yourself are the most important appointments that you have during the next seven days. To highlight this fact, take a highlighter pen and mark these appointments with it.**

Well, we are not naïve enough to assume that just because you highlighted something means that it is going to happen. So consider the following question.

What events are likely to prevent you from keeping the appointments with yourself?

(*Example answers to this question:*
Sleeping late
Dining out
Trip out of town
Fatigue
Laziness)

Now it is your turn.
1....
....
2....
....
3....
....
4....
....
5....
....

The next question to consider is:

How can I make sure that I do what I have promised myself to do?

(Some example answers to this question include:
Setting my alarm clock
Keeping my exercise clothes by my bed
Telling significant others of my plans
Involving others to help me
Cutting out interruptions)

Now it is your turn.

I will not let my goals be jeopardized. To make sure that I meet my goals and overcome barriers I am going to:

1....
....
2....
....
3....
....
4   ....
....
5....
....

Developing Appropriate Boundaries
In order to have time to fit all this good stuff into your schedule you are going to have guard against giving away too much of your time.

How to ensure that you do not get sucked in by other people's demands...

- Do not make an immediate commitment when asked. Always give yourself at least twenty-four hours to consider a request

- Consider where the request fits into your overall priorities

- Consider where is the time going to come from

- Saying no graciously is being gracious, not negative

- You only have yourself to blame if you are over-committed

- If others feel rejected, abandoned and hurt by your *considered, gracious refusal* to comply with their request refer them to a mental health professional.

Having done all this, finalize your seven day goals. You may want to revise them. **You want to set goals that you have an excellent chance of reaching.**

Focusing on your Progress

Now that you have your goals you need to keep track of progress. **It is crucial that you are aware of what you are doing.** To this end you need to keep focused on your daily progress using the Personal HealthScope provided in the back of this book.

The Personal HealthScope helps you keep track of the little dots of your weight management program and at the end of seven days those dots will have formed a bigger picture.

Turn to the Personal HealthScope. You will see that the HealthScope consists of several sections. There is a section on goals in which you circle the labels for eating and exercise behaviors on a daily basis, a review section that you complete on a weekly basis and a section for congratulations and confessions where you can write about your triumphs and disappointments.

Now enter your eating and exercise goals for the next seven days by circling the appropriate labels.

You will see that in the HealthScope there is a section to review your progress every seven days.

The One Person Focus Group

At the end of each seven day period you need to meet with yourself and any other being who might be interested or helpful, like you cat, dog or significant other, and take stock. At this meeting you are going to do the following things.

1. Using your HealthScope, review your eating, exercise and self-care goals for the past week. To what level did you meet your goals?

100%   80%   60%   40%   20%   0%

2. If you met your goals to at least the 60% level, why were you successful?

3. If you met your goals less than 40%, what happened?

4. If you met your goals to the 60% level give yourself a reward.

What rewards are you going to give yourself?
A)
B)
C)

Rewards

Rewards are a way of giving yourself a deserved pat on the back for keeping your commitment to yourself. They are meant to be a token of credit, a symbol of your commitment, not as a materialistic bonanza.

Here are some things that make **good rewards**.

Visit to the beautician
New CD, book or video
Massage
Small, inexpensive item of jewelry or clothing
Tickets (theater not speeding)
Flowers
Cosmetics

Here are some things that are **inappropriate** as rewards

A box of chocolates
A round the world cruise
BMW 935
A new horse

> Never use food as a reward. Rewards are most effective when they are based on **short-term behaviors**, like the goals you set in your Personal HealthScope each week.

    5. Set your eating, exercise and self-care goals for the next seven days. Anticipate the obstacles that might prevent you form doing what you have to do - then deal with them. Be Prepared

    6. If you are cooking, decide exactly when you are doing this and ensure that you have all the items you need.

Now a short test to see if you have been paying attention.

According to Franklin D. Roosevelt, what prevents poor performance?

What technical term did researchers use to describe the factor related to long term success on a behavior change program?[6]

---

[6] *Answers: Perfect planning; Cognitive Vigilance*

Step Three

Mindfulness: Checking Reality

Mindfulness means being aware. It means recognizing that your mind is the single most powerful resource you have to control your actions. This section will provide you with the most powerful strategies there are - not just for managing your weight but controlling your life in general.

The two great principles that govern all behavior are association and repetition. If a reaction becomes associated with an environmental situation it is likely to be repeated. The more it is repeated the more entrenched the behavior becomes. This applies to both physical and mental reactions.

Thinking Habits

Most people think of habits as physical behaviors that are performed. Our most powerful habits, however, are *thinking* habits. Thinking develops in a stylized and habitual way. The foundation of thinking and personality can be traced to the coping skills we developed as young children. Thinking habits develop in childhood. Unless we make a serious attempt to change them as we mature, the chances are that we will continue to react to events from a child's perspective. One definition of maturity is the ability to observe reactions, detach oneself from impulsive desires and thoughts, and evaluate them rationally. This is not easy to do but is the core self-control skill. Many of us are not able to do this and we are stuck responding to situations like threatened children, a state of affairs that prompted Fritz Perls, the famous experiential psychotherapist, to describe adults as "obsolete children."

Consider what happened to this friend of mine. When she was about four, her mother was hospitalized. She remembers being taken to the hospital by her father who, because of his personality and the times (mid 1950's), did not explain to his daughter what was wrong with her mother. My friend was terrified that her mother was going to die. She recalls her anxiety peaking as she approached that hospital. She did not convey this panic to her father because she did not want to burden him just as he was about to lose his wife. (In truth, her mother had just had her appendix removed). She recalls entering the ward where her mother was recovering from her appendectomy. She was immediately whisked away by a nurse into a small playroom while her father disappeared into her mother's room. To this day, my friend will get goose bumps recalling how certain she was that her mother was going to die. So, here she was, in this unfamiliar playroom with this stranger and knowing that her mother was about to die. Imagine what it must have been like for that little girl. Emotionally, she was standing at the peak of terror with enormous clouds of sadness massing on the horizon. Her ears started to ring as her blood pressure soared. She felt a little dizzy. Attention span narrows during times of high anxiety, so all she could see was a rose that has been taken out of an ex-patient's room and placed on a shelf above the rocking horse in the playroom. Her heightened senses imprinted that rose in her nervous system. (She even claims she can smell it to this day.) For a few vital moments the sight and smell of the rose, the hormonal output driving her terror and grief, the physical symptoms of anxiety were all co-mingling to create this unique and very traumatic experience. Somewhere, somehow, in the hundreds of billions of nerve cells that make up the brain and nervous system, this total experience was recorded, captured in memory to forever influence her.

After what seemed like an eternity, the smiling nurse took my friend into her mother's room, where to her complete and utter amazement she found her mother sitting up in bed, looking a little tired but very definitely alive. You can imagine how that little girl rushed to her mother in tears of joy and collapsed on her in total relief. After a few minutes the world returned to normal again: She ate all your mother's grapes, gave her dad a hard time and fell fast asleep on the way home.

A few weeks later her father decided to add some new landscaping to the back yard and triumphantly announced that he has just struck a great deal with the local garden supply business for some beautiful rose bushes. As he revealed a rose specimen, my little friend started to feel dizzy and she began to hyperventilate. She did not know why this was happening but she felt very uncomfortable. She began to cry, telling her father that she hated roses. She was going to leave home if he planted them. Her father interpreted this outburst as another sign that discipline was slack around the house, and while she was in bed lamenting the fact that she missed out on dinner, he was outside planting his new rose bed like a man possessed.

Soon, my friend was avoiding the backyard like the plague, which in a way it was. Whenever she did go into the yard and smell the roses she started to hyperventilate and get wheezy. Her mother, now fully recovered from her appendectomy, noticed these symptoms and duly marched her young daughter off to the local allergist.

This four year old now had a physical and psychological allergy to roses. Thoughts were then created to justify her emotional response. These thinking habits took several forms. *She hated roses. She hated smelly flowers. She vowed never to do any gardening and decided never to even have a backyard.*

Notice that all of these things happened *even though her original anxiety and dread in that waiting room were completely unfounded.* It does not matter that within a few minutes of having that awful experience she was feeling great joy. The fact is that she had the experience, it was recorded and encoded in her nervous system. She had the experience and in the world of psychophysiology *experience is the truth.* Experience is king.

This is a simple example. One environmental cue, a rose, was associated with a very specific reaction. Life is more complex than that. In many situations the traumas are much more subtle and chronic: Parental fights, a drunk father, a mean sibling, a cruel teacher. In many of those situations the reactions are also more subtle but no less powerful and disabling as in my friend's case. Note, too, that in my example the rose was irrelevant, it had nothing to do with the experience except that it happened, by pure chance, to be part of the cue complex associated with a traumatic experience. Note, too, that even if, at a later stage of life, the child had realized the origins of the association, the physical and emotional reactions would not be altered. Knowledge is helpful but often not enough to change the reaction. To change, awareness and ways of managing our consciousness (mindfulness) are needed.[7]

---

[7] My friend now grows beautiful roses. She eventually understood the origin of her fears and deliberately set out to retrain her anxiety by forcing herself to confront roses.

Attitudes about Weight and Food

What has all of this got to do with eating and weight management? Everything. For one thing, where do you think your attitudes about weight or shape or your body originated? I can't tell you the number of clients, almost all women, who have told me that they got their negative views of their bodies from comments made by a significant family member. The comment may have been something like "you're a big girl" or may have referred to some particular part of the anatomy. It may have come from an obsessed parent, a defensive aunt or an obese grandmother. It may have been said in jest, in spite, in fun, in earnest. However it was said, those comments affect you. You take them not only to heart but also deep into your psyche.

Your attitudes and thinking habits about foods were also influenced by the same process. There may well have been a time in your life when ice cream, for example, was associated with positive feelings. When this association occurs you develop thinking habits that reflect this positive association, like "ice cream is good for me," or "ice cream makes me feel better." Suppose it is thirty years later and you are desperately trying to lose weight or trying to fend off diabetes. Is ice cream good for you, now? Will it make you feel better? The answer is no, but unless you are careful, that old thinking habit will prevail. Which brings me to several important rules about thinking habits, growth and maturity.

The Golden Rules of Managing Thinking Habits

Rule number one - most of our thinking habits are adaptive at one point in our lives but eventually they outlive their usefulness. The real trick is to be mindful of those thinking habits that have outlived their usefulness and to change them before they ruin us.

In his classic book, The Road Less Traveled, Scott Peck describes a terrific personal example of what I mean. He describes an evening spent pursuing some quality time with his teenage daughter. They decided to play a game of chess. Peck is a programmed to be somewhat competitive and compulsive. When he plays a game, he plays it to win, no holds barred. Moreover, because he feels that way, he expects his children, including his teenage daughter, to do likewise. So they began to play - and play and play. Time wore on and his daughter lost interest in the game. It was a weeknight and she wanted to prepare for the next school day. Peck would not let the game die. After all, playing a game requires wholehearted commitment. As his daughter encouraged him to hurry his moves, he got more impatient and rigid in his position. "Chess is a serious game. If you're going to play it well, you're going to play it slowly. If you don't want to play it seriously, you might as well not play it at all." They played on for ten minutes until his daughter burst into tears and ran up the stairs sobbing. Which left Scott Peck with the question of how had he got so out of balance. He concluded that his thinking habits, (my words not his), his thinking habit of having to win, of always playing everything so seriously, had outlived its usefulness. It had been very helpful to him as a young boy in school and then as an adult early in his career but now it had got in the way of his being a good father. Peck reports how difficult it was letting go of a habit that had been part of him for such a long time. He got depressed because loss and concession are always depressing. He eventually recovered to appreciate another milestone in his growth. Thinking habits are history and we do have the power to change the future. We are not condemned to live in the past.

Here is the second rule of managing thinking habits. *The more we persist with outmoded thinking habits the more damaging they will be.* One of my clients was a classic perfectionist binger. She was a single woman in her mid-thirties who had spent most of her life obsessed with her weight. She was constantly on a diet and if she did not stick exactly to a demanding nutrition and exercise plan she would become depressed and abandon her program - only to start again a few weeks later with renewed hope and an extra ten pounds. Each time she embarked on the program it was with a determination that this time she would be perfect. There would be no let down - this time she was going to stay with it 100%. Each time she started out doing absolutely everything to perfection - until life intervened - too many social engagements, a viral infection, a sprained ankle, burn-out - and then perfection slipped through her hands and she was left holding jelly doughnuts and cream pies instead. Eventually, she was able to embrace the idea that this pattern was doing more harm than good. Eventually she was able to recognize her rigidity and inability to accept realistic limits. It was not easy, but eventually she was able to learn to control her perfectionist impulses rather than acting them out. By setting herself realistic eating, weight and exercise goals she was able to be successful.

Managing Thoughts and Moods

Managing thoughts is important because thoughts influence moods and behavior. Human beings have an innate tendency to interpret events. They make stories out of what they see. We make assumptions about the events themselves and the motivation that drives them. This tendency to 'write a script' is important to our everyday functioning but it can also get us into big trouble. The biggest problem in relationships is the speed to which we jump to conclusions, often believing them wholeheartedly before we have even checked their validity.

When we write a script it inevitably has our own particular biases imprinted in it. Early in my career, I was working at the University of London's Institute of Psychiatry researching into compulsions and addictions. At that time we were working on a technique called cue exposure which actually forms the basis of some of the temptation management exercises described elsewhere in this program. Early in the development of this technique, I was working with obsessive-compulsive hand washers. These are people who are so afraid of contamination that they spend inordinate amounts of time scrubbing their hands, often so vigorously that they rub the skin right off. Our technique involved exposing them to dirt and then preventing them from washing in the hope that this would extinguish their compulsion. This technique required me to stand in garbage cans. I was demonstrating the fact that nothing terrible happens if you get dirty and don't compulsively wash. One of my clients was in the midst of this retraining program when he decided to take a walk out of the hospital grounds. As he was walking down the road, a garbage truck turned the corner too sharply and dumped a pile of garbage at this poor man's feet. He came storming into the hospital and at the first opportunity accosted me vigorously. "I saw you driving that garbage truck, Dr. Rankin," he accused. Of course, I was not, but he had written his script and had assumed that I was simply giving him another test.

We assume that our own thoughts and interpretations, particularly about other people's behavior, are accurate without subjecting them to any sort of reality check. One of the best examples of this is provided by Dave Barry in his amusing and perceptive book, Dave Barry's Complete Guide to Guys (Random House, New York, 1995). In it, he describes a typical conversation that says a lot about gender differences in communication as well as our tendency to believe our own script. The
62

conversation between Elaine and Roger as they are heading home in the car goes something like this.

Elaine opens the conversation by commenting that it is six months since they started dating. After a short while Roger realizes, within the confines of the privacy of his own mind, that his means that they started dating in February, which was the last time the car was in the dealers for an oil change, which means that, hey, his car is way overdue for an oil change.

Elaine can see the change in Roger's demeanor and assumes that he is upset with her. She assumes he must be upset because he wants more commitment and more intimacy. She reaches this conclusion on the basis of nothing but her own wishes. Meanwhile, back in Roger's head there is more action. He is deep in thought about the transmission. The car is still not shifting right and the morons at the garage better see to it this time. He is getting really angry thinking about this and Elaine can see it.

Elaine now feels guilty for putting him through all of this and even mentioning the relationship in the first place. Meanwhile Roger is thinking about the excuses the garage are going to give him and what he's going to do to them. And Elaine continues with her existential crisis while Roger continues with his automotive crisis and the two never quite meet.

What Dave Barry is so brilliantly and so amusingly describing is our tendency to believe our own propaganda without ever checking its validity. I have used this particular passage in particular and "Dave Barry's Complete Guide to Guys" in general with many couples that come to me for counseling.

Automatic Thinking

We get into situations and our thinking becomes automatic. Automatic thoughts trigger automatic moods and before we know it we are off beam, off base and off track.

A participant in one of my seminars described the following experience. She had been on the program for a few days and was feeling really good. She had started an exercise program and had regained control of her eating. After lunch she decided to take a walk. She set out feeling very good. She was enjoying walking, listening to the birds, feeling good with no interest in eating at all. Food was the farthest thing from her mind.

As she progressed on her walk she passed two people eating her favorite candy bar. As she saw the wrapper the first thing that entered her mind was "It would be great to have one of those right now." The next automatic thought was, "Isn't it a shame that I cannot eat one." Then it was "it's unfair that I cannot eat one." As she looked out at the street she thought to herself, "Look at all these lucky people - they can eat all the candy they want but I can't. I am fed up with battling this problem. It's dogged me all of my life. It's not fair and I am fed up with it." Obviously if those are the thoughts that are passing through your mind, you do not feel very good and this woman reported that, whereas she had been feeling on top of the world she was now feeling very dispirited. Her mood had changed in matter of seconds. A mild desire for a candy bar had turned into an existential crisis.

If this woman had not taken control of her mind and managed her thoughts there was a very real danger that she would have soon found herself in the store buying at least one, probably more, of her favorite candy bars. Fortunately, she was able to intervene and say to herself the following. "Wait a second. I used to think like that. That candy bar will only make me feel good for a very short time, after that I will feel terrible. Besides, I don't need a candy bar right now - or even want one. This is just an old tape playing and I don't have to listen. I have done well on this program and I am feeling great."

This woman was able to practice mindfulness and it prevented her from relapsing.

In the temptation management phase of this program there are exercises designed to help you challenge some of your thinking habits about food and temptation in particular. But what can you do to change your destructive thinking habits?

Changing Destructive Thinking Habits

Recognizing damaging thinking habits is the first step. The are various categories of thinking habits and I have identified ones that are relevant to losing weight and present the greatest barriers to proper self-care.

The first of these stems from perfectionism. There is nothing wrong with trying to be perfect as long as you recognize that aiming for it and achieving it are two quite different things. Human beings are not perfect. They have limitations and imperfections. Because you are a human being you are not perfect either. The danger with perfectionism is that it inhibits ambition through fear of failure. It also leads to premature abandonment of a program when obstacles and difficulties arise.

Success is gained by perseverance not perfectionism. The perfectionist's thinking habits are likely to be very self-defeating. Their criteria for success are very strict and their goals often unrealistic. The perfectionist will not give themselves credit for making an effort or even meeting a goal. The perfectionist will find it difficult to accept credit or praise from another person. The perfectionist will believe that anything less than 100% all of the time is tantamount to failure. The perfectionist will beat themselves up if they do not meet their high goals exactly and even if they do meet them, they will still be unhappy. The perfectionist will start to feel uncomfortable if they deviate from their goals and are likely to abandon them altogether on the assumption that they will never be reached

What the perfectionist has to learn to do is to harness their compulsive drive for high standards and temper it within reasonable limits. You are not going to stick to your plan every day. You are not going to do it 100% of the time, all the time. But if you do it enough of the time, it will make a difference. You might even get to enjoy it. The perfectionist needs to lighten up - to allow herself some treats now and then and consider the big picture not the minor details of the here and now.

Other Worries

The compulsive worrier is a person who constantly anticipates the worst. While being prepared is helpful, even necessary, spending time and energy over things that will probably never happen is not a useful strategy. As one of my clients once said to me, "I have had many problems in my life and some of them have actually happened."

All of us are likely at times to sink into old thinking habits and view the world negatively. There is a direct relationship between energy and positive thinking. The more positive you are, the more energy you have and vice-versa. States like hunger, frustration and fatigue which drain energy elicit more negative thinking habits. That is one reason why it is not a good idea to embark on a sensitive discussion after about nine o'clock at night. It is more difficult to be rational and tolerant when you are out of energy. At times of low energy, more vigilance is required to prevent negativity.

Negative thoughts need to be challenged. Like the woman in the candy bar example mentioned above, you need to stand back and conduct a thorough reality check.

The most effective and adaptive outlook is to keep a positive spin on events. This does not require you to be a Pollyanna and pretend everything is rosy when it is not. It does mean that you seek wherever possible, to find positive value and meaning in your life circumstances. Coping is about finding positive meaning.

Studies of patients suffering from serious illnesses often show that a positive attitude is associated with better coping and better survival rates. A classic study conducted in London rated people with cancer according to their attitude and outlook. There were three groups: those who were very positive and kept their life going despite their illness, those who basically denied the illness and those who became consumed by their illness and its treatment. Survival rates were best for the positive thinkers, next best for the deniers and worst for those who were consumed by their condition.

It is perfectly reasonable for someone to become consumed by their illness, especially if its serious. However, such an attitude while understandable and logical, may not be very adaptive. *Adaptation* is the key word, here. Human beings thrive and survive when they cope and adapt. Finding positive meaning in your life is the most adaptive for you, even if it does not reflect some objective truth. If you believe it - it can be helpful.

66

The Positive Spin

I can not give you a magic formula for putting a positive spin on the events in your life. However, I can give you some ways of preventing negative thoughts and some tools for helping you develop a more positive attitude. You will find these tools in the exercises that follow.

One of these tools involves learning how to stand back from your thoughts and not automatically embrace them. This skill is essential if you are going to be a good reality checker. Simple meditation techniques help the development of this skill and these are included in the exercises follow.

Other exercises include useful reality checkers, ways of identifying outmoded thinking habits, particularly in relation to food, eating and weight. There are also tips on how to manage high levels of emotion. One of these is a technique for monitoring your thoughts for extremes - the "always" and the "nevers" that creep into your thoughts.

How many times have you cruised the parking lot looking for the perfect parking space? Sometimes you find one and sometimes you don't. If you just happen to miss one, however, you will probably say to yourself "That always happens to me, I always just miss out." Depending on your frustration tolerance you will either continue to circle the parking lot looking for the ultimate space, take the handicap space or burn rubber tearing out of the lot in complete frustration. It does not always happen to you, you do not always miss out - it just feels like it does. If you accept that thinking, however, frustration won't be far behind.

The exercises will also identify the dangers of accepting moral imperatives - words like "ought" and "should" that can create similar havoc on thoughts, moods and behaviors.

These tools are all keys to a healthy mental life as well as a healthy lifestyle, so please make sure you read the exercises and practice them.

Developing Awareness

In order to manage your thinking you need to:

1. Identify toxic thoughts and flush them away
2. Rewrite old thinking habits so that they are more adaptive
3. Master the art of the reality check and learn how to manage thoughts

Identifying Toxic Thoughts

Toxic thoughts are those ideas that are unhelpful to you and lead you into uncomfortable feelings and destructive behaviors. You can have toxic thoughts about anything, not just food, your eating and your weight. Toxic thoughts fall into the following categories.

Thoughts that get you into trouble.
For example: I *need* that cheesecake

Thoughts that are expressed as extremes
For example: I *never* get what I want

Thoughts that imply obligation
For example: I *must* eat this otherwise I will appear rude to my host

Thoughts that are associated with unhelpful behaviors
For example: A binge will make me feel better

Thoughts lead to feelings and feelings lead to behavior

Answer the following questions.

What do you think your favorite foods do for you?

....

....

What do you think about your weight management and wellness efforts?

....

....

What do you think about your chances of maintaining a healthy lifestyle?

....

....

Now I want you to ask yourself, how realistic have you been in that last exercise? Are these ideas merely old thinking habits or do they accurately reflect the current state of affairs?

Ways of Turning Old Thinking Habits Into More Positive Ideas.

Some thinking habits need to be discarded completely, others can be rewritten. For example, suppose you have written this about your favorite foods.

I love cheesecake. It always makes me feel good and it always tastes wonderful. I cannot imagine ever resisting it. These ideas need to be revised

Old thinking habit	Rewritten thought
I love cheesecake.	*I enjoy eating cheesecake*
It always makes me feel good.	*I like the taste*
It always tastes wonderful.	*Some cheesecake is better than others*
I cannot imagine resisting it.	*I can live without it*

Then we need to add..
I don't like the long term effects of the fat
Sometimes I regret having eaten it

By rewriting the thought you have a more balanced, helpful and more adaptive view of your relationship with cheesecake.

Whenever the old thinking habits resurface in your mind, you have to flush them away. Using the motivational link method learn to see and hear yourself flushing away these toxic, unhelpful thinking habits.

Consider another example. Suppose you have the following thought:

"I have tried many programs in the past which have never worked and this won't be any different. I'll probably do this for a short while and then I'll give up. I have to lose weight but I think I am destined to always be overweight."

If you analyze the above you will see it contains several toxic elements.

Toxic thought
This program won't work
I will give up after a short while
I have to lose weight
I am destined to be overweight

Rewrite the script above, discarding the toxic thoughts and replacing them with more adaptive ideas.

Some suggestions	
Toxic thought	Adaptive thought
This program won't work	I am going to try my best with this
I will give up after a short while	I will take it one day at a time
I have to lose weight	I chose to try to lose weight
I am destined to be overweight	I have the power to get control of my weight

Now rewrite your thoughts and ideas about food, eating, your weight and your body so that they are more adaptive.

Food:
....
....
....

Eating:
....
....
....

My Weight:

....

....

....

My Body:

....

....

....

Mastering the Art of the Reality Check

Here are some questions you can ask yourself to determine whether your thinking is realistic or simply a toxic thought.

Do you always think the same way?
Is this a negative or a positive thought?
Is the verb in the thought a positive or negative one?
Does the thought contain the words "always" or "never"?
Does the thought contain a sense of obligation conveyed by such words as "ought" and "must"?
Does the thought contain the idea that you have a choice?
Does the thought contain the idea that you have power?
What would you say to a friend who expressed the same idea?

Remember: Just because an idea is passing through your head does not make it true, valid or acceptable. You have the power to monitor your thoughts and manage them effectively.

Meditation

One secret to the practice of mindfulness is the ability to detach from intrusive thoughts. Such detachment makes objectivity more likely. The following exercises contain ways of practicing detachment.

The mind filters out an enormous amount of incoming stimulation. It does this to prevent being overwhelmed by the continuous bombardment of sensory input. Our consciousness can only attend to one input at a time. Our ability to switch attention rapidly creates the illusion that we can attend to several inputs simultaneously. The exercises that follow will help you get some control of that attentional filter which in turn will help you manage thoughts more effectively.

Blank mind

Try to blank your mind. Close your eyes and try to think of nothing for the next minute.

What happened? Almost inevitably you found that after a short while you found thoughts intruding into your consciousness. You probably started to engage those thoughts and before long were engrossed in them. Stopping the process of being distracted by passing thoughts typically takes much practice.

Meditation is not necessarily above having a blank mind. Meditation can help you learn how to redirect attention and ultimately gain control over thoughts.

In this next exercise, rather than trying to keep your mind blank, try to concentrate on something specific. Just follow the simple instructions.

Breath Focus

Breathing in through your nose, take a slow, deep, controlled breath. Exhale slowly by blowing out through your mouth. Inhale again, slowly through your mouth. Exhale, slowly by blowing out through your mouth. Keep it going. Inhale slowly, exhale slowly. Inhale slowly, exhale slowly. As you are doing this just concentrate on the sound of the air going in and out of your body.

What happened this time? You may have found it easier not to get distracted by intruding thoughts because you were focused on your breathing. Here is another exercise.

Movie screen

Imagine a big movie screen, like you would find at a drive-in theater. The words "my weight" are written in big letters in the middle of the movie screen. Imagine that the words "my weight" are on that movie screen. Just keep focused on the words - keep you eyes glued to that movie screen. Keep focused on the words "my weight." Now watch the words move to the left and the letters disappear off the end of the screen - one by one until there is nothing on the screen any more.

Hopefully you were able to find yourself distancing yourself from the emotional content of the thought by simply viewing it as an objective presence on the screen. If you did not - do not worry. Practice will help you do this.

River bank

Imagine that you are sitting on a river bank. The river is below you. It flows from your right, passes in front of you and then curves to the left out of sight behind an island of trees. You're sitting on the river bank on a warm spring day. There's a gentle breeze blowing in your hair and you can feel the warmth of the sunshine on your face. As you watch the river, you can see the thought "I feel good" emerging from the right - floating on the river. Watch it as it slowly floats past you, off to the left and slowly disappears around the island of trees and out of sight.

River bank: Self-generated thought

Now as you sit there on that river bank, take the first thought that comes to mind and watch it float slowly on that river. See it start out from the right and float slowly past you and then watch it as it curves left past the island of trees and out of sight.

These skills take practice. The more you repeat them, however, the more they will help you control your thinking.

Now a short test to see if you have been paying attention.

1. **What is the technical name given to the habit of jumping to your own conclusions before adequate reality testing?**

2. **Who wrote "The Guide to Guys"?[8]**

---

[8] Answers: Projection: Dave Barry

Step Four

Binge Management: Defusing The Bomb

Bingeing is one of the most destructive eating habits. Thousands of calories, often high in fat, are consumed very quickly during a binge. Millions of people have this problem which causes physical and psychological distress as well as weight problems. How is a binge defined and what is the treatment for this condition?

Until recently, bingeing was considered only as part of bulimia, an eating disorder that involves self-induced vomiting and excessive laxative use. It is now recognized that bingeing without purging or laxative use, is a very common behavior. Bingeing is common in both men and women and is distressing on a number of counts. Physically, it can lead to rapid weight gain and wildly fluctuating weight. Psychologically, it is associated with feelings of shame, guilt, disgust and lack of control. Although both men and women admit to bingeing, a recent study conducted by myself and my colleagues at the University of South Carolina, found that men were less distressed by the consequences of bingeing.[9]

What is a Binge?

The emotional significance of a binge is often greater than the caloric one. Cultural, gender and individual differences can mean that one person's binge is another person's snack. Consequently, the definition of a binge has focused more on the psychological, rather than the caloric aspects. Consequently, the number of calories consumed is not an adequate measure of a binge. One cookie might send a ballerina into paroxysms of anxiety whereas a whole box of cookies might not bother a truck driver.

The emotional reactions to a binge have become the central focus for the definition. Feelings of disgust and lack of control after eating are the two main criteria. These uncomfortable feelings are determined by many factors, including high self-expectations and rigid goals.

---

[9] DiGiacchino, R., Sargent, R., Rankin, H., Streeter, S and Sharpe, P, (1998) submitted for publication

74

Bingeing is destructive physically because human beings have a capacity to rapidly consume hundreds of calories. The average time to consume a meal of burger, fries and milk-shake - about 1200 calories - is four and a half minutes! The bulimics that were treated on my eating disorders in England, typically reported binges of between three thousand and ten thousand calories, often eaten in less than half-an-hour. Dr. Gerald Russell, former colleague and one of the world's foremost eating disorders specialists, told me of a client who confessed to a 70,000 calorie binge. The consumption of large amounts of calories is obviously not conducive to successful weight maintenance or wellness.

A binge typically has a compulsive element to it. Often the urge to eat feels uncontrollable, which has led some to believe that there is a physiological basis to the behavior. Evidence suggests that *some* bingeing may be physiologically driven. This has led to the development of medications that are designed to reduce the bingeing urge. Some of these medications have been shown to have serious side-effects and have been withdrawn from the market. Other drugs have not been subject to long-term clinical trials. Be aware, therefore. that the currently available medications are not panaceas. Theoretically, drugs may help moderate your compulsive drive but they will not fundamentally change your thoughts and behaviors. Medications can theoretically be useful if they relieve the physical compulsion and *you take advantage of that fact to make the necessary behavioral and psychological changes*. Medications themselves, however, are not a substitute for behavior change methods. For example, even before some of these drugs were shown to have serious physical side-effects, this is what the The Pocket PDR 1996 edition, said about Phentermine, a drug you might know it as Fastin or Ionamin:

" Always remember that Fastin is an aid to, not a substitute for, good diet and exercise. Fastin should be used along with a behavior modification program. Take Fastin only as directed by your doctor. Do not take it more often or for a longer time than your doctor has ordered. Fastin can lose its effectiveness after a few weeks."[10]

---

[10] The PDR Pocket Guide to Prescription Drugs, Pocket Books, New York, 1996

In short, this medication, like many others in the mental health field, is not a substitute for change, but it can make it more likely that you will do the things necessary to effect change.

Binge Dynamics

When you binge, you not only eat fast food but you eat it fast. You abandon the formal rules of dining etiquette and bingeing is often done on the run, or standing up or while doing some other activity. If you are a binger, you should try, wherever possible, to only eat when sitting down. Slowing your eating and being deliberate is a useful tactic, too. However, these behavioral tactics are often not immediately manageable for the seasoned binger.

Moreover, a binge is almost always done on one's own in complete privacy. This most likely will be done within the confines of your own home, especially in your own room or even in your own closet.

In one of my seminars, a CEO of a mid-sized company, admitted that on some occasions, she would return from a busy day at the office, make herself a peanut butter and jelly sandwich and eat it. Nothing strange about that you may think, except that once she had made the sandwich, she locked herself in a closet until she had finished it. This is a successful, intelligent woman although these actions do not suggest it. Why did she act like this and what does this tell us about bingeing? I'll answer that question shortly.

The car is also a popular place to binge. I have many clients who have told me that the car is the most common place to binge. One client of mine used to take her lunch break, simply stuffing the food in her mouth as she drove from one fast food place to another.

The bedroom is also another popular place to binge, especially when alone. Such behavior suggests a link between loneliness, lack of intimacy and bingeing.

Bingeing is also done privately because it is associated with great guilt and shame. Where does that guilt and shame originate?

Guilt and Shame

Some bingers confess to shame about eating anything. This shame can be associated with childhood experiences in which the eating of treats was considered sinful. Often, these bingers grew up with controlling, restrictive and punitive parents who had a vendetta against indulgence. Such an environment leads children to sneak foods and to feel great guilt for natural desires.

Parents can be very cruel and critical of a child's weight. Such parents are obsessed with weight and diet and can literally give their offspring a neurosis about their eating, their weight ands themselves. Parental guilt trips and dire warnings about weight lead bingers to have unrealistic and frankly irrational views about her relationship between their eating, their weight and themselves. While bingeing on high fat foods is detrimental to weight, some bingers overreact often believing that a one hundred calorie cookie will immediately add pounds to their hips.[11]

One of my clients told me the following story about her childhood. Her mother was very obsessive about both her own weight and that of her daughter, my client. It is apparent that her mother had been anorexic and she imposed severe food restrictions on her children. She constantly warned her daughter about the evils of overweight. She was so obsessive about food that her daughter frequently went without proper nutrition. This meant that the young child was hungry and she resorted to sneaking into the kitchen late at night. This made her feel guilty, ashamed and also afraid of being caught. This child was not sneaking candies, ice-cream, or other treats as much as she would love to eat them. She was "sneaking" plain bread and cereal. As a result, guilt, shame and fear became associated with eating. When the girl grew up and was free of her mother's tyranny, she started bingeing heavily which only reinforced her shame, guilt and anxiety. Clarifying the obvious dynamics of her was not sufficient to control the bingeing habit. She had to learn how to

---

[11] I know it *feels* like that but the math does not add up. Even if 100 calories was immediately metabolized that way, 15% of the calories would be used in digestion. Given that there are 3500 calories in a pound, even if the 85 calories left did go straight to your hips (and they don't) the maximum gain would be about 0.4 of an ounce!

eat without these uncomfortable feelings and this required psychological and behavioral reprogramming. which utilized the mindfulness exercises that are included with this program. Such a technique empowers you to manage destructive thoughts. The behavioral reprogramming involves learning to experience eating without the associated shame, guilt and fear. The implication of this reprogramming is that if you chose to eat something you should eat it and enjoy it. Don't second guess yourself. Do not be ashamed or guilty. You have a perfect right to eat whatever you choose. The exercises in this chapter include learning to eat some of your favorite foods without shame, fear and guilt.

Expectations

I have had good success treating bingers and bulimics by helping them change their unrealistic expectations and savagely high standards. In my experience, perfectionism and control issues are rife amongst bingers. They are often people who have unrealistic goals. When they cannot meet these goals, panic increases, igniting a vicious spiral of failure set off by their own high standards. The higher the standards the likelier the failure, the greater the panic, the more the bingeing.

Because of these perfectionism and control issues, bingers are often all-or-nothing thinkers and doers. If you are like this, you know that you will follow your program perfectly for a few days but then get easily deflected. The slide begins when you have twelve hundred calories instead of eleven hundred, or eat a frozen yogurt that you had not planned. This feels like failure and within a short space of time your program has vanished, It has probably gone into reverse with eating completely out of control.

One of my former clients was a highly intelligent girl - she was studying for her Ph.D. in one of Britain's most prestigious universities - who was referred to my unit after she had eaten her way through a freezer filled with food for a family of six for the upcoming holidays. Her family did not know what more they could do with her. They were at their wits end. She was one of the most perfectionistic and tightly controlled people I have ever met. She was so insistent on control that she needed to be mildly sedated just to keep her in the hospital. Despite the fact the unit was run in a non-threatening way, this girl fought every inch of the way. On her second night in the hospital, she broke into the kitchen and drank all of the milk that she could find - a staggering 26 pints of it! (she was only 4'10"). She needed to control everything and if she felt she wasn't able to do that - she panicked and ate. Eventually we were, in the confines of a controlled environment, able to get her to trust us enough to begin to feel comfortable without having total control. She was gradually able to let go and learn to control her bingeing.

Another patient was the classic yo-yo dieter. She was obsessed with perfection. She panicked if she thought she had even one hair out of place. Everything she did had to meet the most exacting criteria. Imagine how tiring, not to mention tiresome, that is. When she felt in control, she was being upbeat and functional. When she felt she wasn't in control, she binged heavily and became very depressed. Depression deepened when she realized that the idea of total control is a complete fantasy. In this case, bingeing was the result of the failure to meet high standards. Once you have violated a goal there is a natural tendency to abandon it altogether. Alan Marlatt, a leading addictions psychologist, coined the phrase "abstinence violation effect" to describe this phenomena. He observed that once addicts violated their abstinence, they would give up trying to exert any semblance of control.

The woman in the above example also used bingeing to medicate her panic. Frequently, bingeing is used to numb the pain of frustration, rejection and emptiness and to temper the extremes of anxiety and anger.

Controlling Emotions
Bingeing creates several physical feelings that help blot out the discomfort of emotions. Numbing feelings with food might be more appealing than doing it with alcohol and drugs because those substances might make you feel really out of control. It is not surprising, however, that many bulimics and bingers also have problems with alcohol.

Bingeing creates the feeling of fullness. Fullness is associated with the primitive security of having a full stomach. At a primitive level hunger is associated with fears of survival, fullness associated with feelings of security. At a more sophisticated level, many bingers report feelings of spiritual emptiness that trigger bingeing. Physical fullness is an unsatisfactory way of compensating for spiritual emptiness.

Bingeing can also create a feeling of nausea, which at least is more manageable than anger, frustration or boredom. Because of its primitive and urgent nature, nausea has the virtue of distracting you from other feelings.

Numbness, caused by high sugar intake, often follows a binge. Sugar gives you a buzz in the short term but numbs you out thereafter. Sugar influences brain chemistry thus altering your experience of emotions.

The feelings that are most associated with bingeing are anger, frustration, loneliness and depression.

Anger is an uncomfortable state that can be mistaken for anxiety. With both anger and anxiety there is an increase in sympathetic nervous system arousal which sets up the fight or flight response. Anger can result in increased heart rate and adrenaline, leading to a sense of loss of control.

All emotions are the result of social perceptions. Anger occurs on the perception of unfair treatment. As well as increased physiological arousal, guilt and denial often accompany anger. Many people are trained by their parents that anger is wrong and they thus confuse their emotions with their morals. Feeling angry is no more wrong than a headache is wrong. Like a headache, anger is uncomfortable, but it is not a moral sin. The invalidation of anger is one of the leading causes of psychological distress. It can lead to depression, violence, addiction, panic and bingeing.

The yo-yo dieter mentioned above, was raised in an angry environment. Children do not have the mental and psychological resources to deal effectively with difficult emotions. Her coping strategy was to become a peacemaker. She thought that if she was perfect she could control her parents' anger and chaos. Unless a child is specifically informed to the contrary, it assumes that she or he is responsible for parental emotions, especially anger. This child was no exception and firmly believed that she was responsible for all of the family dynamics, including the anger. She really believed her perfection would resolve the family problems. This perfectionistic policy never works and reinforces the child's belief that they are responsible for the family difficulties. The solution is always to try harder rather than
80

abandon the impossible. This puts a terrific burden on the child who thus develops the thinking habit that all anger is bad and should be suppressed at all costs. Moreover, she will also feel a tremendous responsibility to be perfect in order to control the emotions of others. The imperfect becomes unacceptable and this creates enormous anxiety for the young child who has few resources to relieve such discomfort. Food is an available comforter, however, so it is hardly surprising that sweets and treats in particular become valued as way of coping.

Ego States

We are creatures of many moods and different ego-states. An ego state is a state of mind characterized by certain feelings, thoughts and behaviors that exist together as a sensory complex, which I call ego-state packages or ESP's. The concept of multiple ego-states is best seen in those with multiple personality disorder. In this condition it isn't the multiplicity of ego-states that is abnormal but the fragmentation and separation of those states that characterizes the disorder. All of us have multiple sides to our personality, but we have a sense of integration. Our different ego states are connected in a way that is not apparent in MPD. Multiple Personality Disorder has recently been renamed Dissociative Identity Disorder (DID) to reflect the new clinical emphasis on fragmentation rather than multiplicity.

DID is a dissociative disorder. Dissociation reflects an ability to psychologically detach from the immediate environment. Dissociation is a continuous concept with pathological dissociation like DID at one end of the continuum, and normal dissociation, like highway hypnosis, at the other. In highway hypnosis you suddenly realize that you are unaware of driving the last few miles. You were so deep in thought that it seemed as if you were not actually driving. You were driving, of course, and probably quite safely. You were on auto-pilot or using today's terminology, you were multi-tasking - doing two things at once - driving and contemplating. Because you can only have one focus to your consciousness at any one time you may be doing something else, like driving or indeed bingeing, but not be aware of doing it. Dissociation, doing an activity on autopilot while not attending to what you are doing, is very common during bingeing. For example, have you ever eaten food and realized that you never even tasted it?. Or have you eaten and lost track of how much you have eaten? Or have you been aware of having eaten but can't remember exactly what it was that you ate?

People dissociate while they are eating in different ways. Some people read while eating, others watch television and others get engrossed in conversation. All of these activities distract attention from what is being eaten. There are various reasons for diverting attention in this way. Avoidance of guilt, shame and other unpleasant feelings is one reason. Denial of the fact that what one is eating is inconsistent with a stated wellness goal, is another. A third reason is the sheer habit of not attending and diverting awareness from eating behavior.

Awareness of your eating is crucial. You can not learn to control a behavior that you are ignoring. Increasing awareness of eating involves disconnecting it from other activities. When you are eating it should be the main activity and command full attention. These and other tactics are described in the exercises that accompany this chapter.

Let's suppose you have an ego-state package that involves bingeing. In certain situations, this ego state will be triggered and you will play out a set of thoughts, feelings and behaviors that include bingeing. This ego-state was probably derived in childhood in response to certain emotional and interpersonal conditions. If those conditions arise, the ego-state is activated and all of the feelings and compulsions associated with a binge will be triggered. Your logical present mind will make an attempt to maintain control but the binge package is powerful and can temporarily overwhelm logic. Once that binge ego-state has played out, you return to a more rational state. At that point you may feel guilt and shame and are frustrated by your lack of control.

That is why the CEO mentioned earlier is sitting in the closet eating PBJ sandwiches. Or why the woman is spending her lunch time driving from fast food place to fast food place. Their ESP's are somehow triggered and they "find" themselves indulging in behavior that is definitely not part of their rational plan. Many of my clients report finding themselves at the refrigerator, pulling out the ice -cream, but not really remembering much about the decision to get there - it's as if they have been beamed to the freezer by Scotty from Star Trek. How do you learn to manage ego-states that influence your behavior in such a destructive way?

First, it is important to understand the dynamics of this behavior and the exercises that accompany this section will help you do just that. Then you need to identify the different elements of the ego-state and when it occurs. Then skills and preventive strategies that control the ego-state need to be developed. Two important ways of defusing these ego-states involve physical activity and sharing. These two activities keep you anchored in a more rational state and will help in your binge control.

Bingeing can be brought under control. The retraining exercises that follow will help you reduce your extremism both in your perfectionism and your control. In other words - lighten up! The behavioral exercises that follow will help you learn to eat without shame, guilt and fear.

In addition, the exercises that follow also provide tools for helping you manage emotional eating. As you have already seen, managing your emotions, especially frustration, anger and emptiness, is key to controlling binge eating.

Controlling Bingeing, Emotional Eating and Stress

Any behavior that is used to control emotions will become compulsive. Eating to reduce unpleasant feelings is no exception. Such emotional eating will quickly become compulsive as well as impulsive and unplanned. It will also become automatic.

Unconscious Eating

Have you ever eaten food, and afterwards not been aware of how much you have eaten?

Have you eaten food and realized that you were not even aware of tasting it?

Have you had a vague awareness of having eaten something within a couple of hours but can not remember what it was?

An emotional eater will also find it hard to resist food. If they can resist, they often obsess about it endlessly.

The problem with bingeing and emotional eating is that it is very destructive to both the eater's *weight control efforts and their state of mind.*

There are three keys to managing emotional eating and thus giving yourself a realistic chance at controlling your weight.

These three keys are:

1. Changing your eating habits and associations with food

2. Changing your response to frustration, anger, emptiness, depression and tension - the main emotions responsible for binge eating

3. Changing distorted thinking and unrealistic expectations

Changing Eating Habits and Associations
Throughout this program, I have stressed the importance of associations and repetition, and I have used these principles to help you establish new behaviors. Association and repetition, however, have also created problems for you if you are an emotional eater.

Imagine a situation in which feelings of loneliness are a trigger (or cue) for eating. Let's suppose that along the way you have developed a habit of eating whenever feelings of loneliness flash through your consciousness. Let us suppose that when you get these feelings you go into the kitchen and make yourself two large peanut butter sandwiches. Let us also suppose that immediately after you have eaten these two sandwiches (about 700 calories) you feel comforted for about five minutes. After that time, you feel somewhat frustrated with yourself for doing this when a few hours earlier you vowed to stop the habit for good. After about ten minutes, you are feeling disgusted and very angry with yourself. Anger is a difficult emotion to handle, and as such is cue for further eating. There is a good chance that eating might resume in response to the anger and disgust accompanied by an appropriate rationalization ("What's the point, I've started now," "I'll start again tomorrow") to justify your actions.

This cycle is vicious and uncompromising. Let's consider the associations that have been created with this habit.

Loneliness & Food (peanut butter sandwiches)
Loneliness & Disgust
Loneliness & Self-hate
Food & Comfort
Food & Disgust
Food & Self-hate
Food & Anger
Comfort & Anger

It is not difficult to see why you might be so emotional about your eating - and confused.

It gets more complicated. The more entrenched this habit becomes the more powerful the associations are. What may have started out as eating in response to major feelings of loneliness may now occur if you are just a little bored. It might well get to the point when even the *anticipation* of possible loneliness will stimulate cravings for peanut butter sandwiches. You may find yourself eating without a conscious reason. After a while the cues associated with this habit, including loneliness, the sight of peanut butter, even your kitchen wallpaper, can produce strong cravings..

What you have to do to break this eating cycle is to *disassociate these cues from your behavior and defuse them of the power that they have over you.*

Defuse the Cues!

First, you need to identify the cues that exert power over you. Cues to binge can be emotions, thoughts, places, people, even times of day. What are your cues? Check the appropriate column for each of the common cues that are listed in the box.

	Hardly Ever	Sometimes	Always
I binge when I feel angry			
I binge when I feel depressed			
I binge when I feel frustrated			
I binge when I feel tense			
I binge when I feel sad			
I binge when I feel happy			
I binge when I feel lonely			
I binge when I feel guilty			
I binge when I am at work			
I binge when I am in my bedroom			
I binge when I am in my living room			
I binge when I am in the bathroom			
I binge in the morning			
I binge in the middle of the afternoon			
I binge in the early evening			
I binge late at night			
I binge when I am on my own			

Other binge cues are:

My favorite binge foods are:

Now you have identified those situations that cue a binge, you need to find ways of dealing with them other than bingeing.

Ego-States
As I mentioned earlier, bingeing often occurs as part of an ego-state package of specific thoughts, feelings and behaviors. What thoughts, feelings and other behaviors typically accompany a binge?

Thoughts that immediately precede a binge:
....
....
....

Thoughts that accompany a binge:

....

....

....

Thoughts that follow a binge:

....

....

....

Feelings that immediately precede a binge:

....

....

....

Feelings that follow a binge:

....

....

....

Cue Preparedness

Prepare to handle these situations as they arise by generating a list of possible alternative actions (other than eating) that could be taken.

Alternatives to bingeing
Call a friend
Read a book
Watch TV
Go to the mall
Do yard work
Go to the movies
Do paperwork
Play your favorite music
Visit a friend
Walk the dog
Do a puzzle
Meditate/relax
Listen to the radio
Ride your bike

Now, make your own coping list. Consider activities that you could do:

⇒ In your home

⇒ Outside the home (e.g. movies, friends' homes, the Mall etc.)

⇒ On your own

⇒ With other people

Tip: Whatever else you do, pour yourself a glass of water first and drink it. That will buy you some precious time and will also help fill you up.

Keep your list in front of you at all times. Practice your coping strategies.

The more practiced your coping strategies are, the better off you will be.

Next, let us use the power of your imagination.

Imagery exercise: Imagine yourself facing a situation which normally cues a binge. Only this time, imagine successfully resisting the binge by doing an alternative activity like the ones described above. Imagine not eating at all. Feel the power.

As you disassociate food and emotional eating it may be possible, if you wish, to eat your usual binge foods in moderation. *The secret to this is not to eat them in response to emotional cues.* Using the loneliness/peanut butter sandwich example described above, you may get to a point when you can, occasionally, have a peanut butter sandwich. This would *never be eaten as a response to an emotion, only as a treat when you were feeling content.*[12]

---

[12]Once you have disassociated your binge foods from the cues that trigger them you may never want to eat them again.

88

Managing Anger, Frustration, Emptiness, Depression and Tension

The most common emotions associated with binge eating are anger, frustration, emptiness, depression and tension.

Frustration, occurs when you are thwarted in an attempt to reach your goals and realize your expectations. Bingers as a group tend to be perfectionistic and often have unrealistic expectations, which, in turn, sets them up for frustration.

Anger comes when you perceive you have been treated unfairly. Many people believe that to be angry is somehow wrong or immoral. Anger is a perfectly normal human emotion. Anger is not the same as hate - although it sometimes feels as if it is.

Frustration often feels like anger. One big difference between the two is that when you are angry you have an object to your anger and when you are frustrated you do not. Frustration occurs when there really is no-one to blame, unlike anger where there is a very definite person responsible for your injustice.

Managing Anger and Frustration

Validation. It is not the feeling of anger that is the potential problem - it is how it is managed. You need to accept your anger, recognize its strong points and manage it effectively.

Anger and Love, It is possible to be angry with someone you love. Anger and love are not incompatible, although it is tough to feel them simultaneously.

Anger as Self-expression. Anger is the ultimate self-expression. It is standing up for what you perceive to be an injustice and thus the feeling of anger and its appropriate expression is an important component of self-esteem.

Specific tactics for handling anger include:

Time Out: Do not act impulsively. Give yourself a chance to cool down by taking a time-out. That often means physically leaving a situation. Time provides a great perspective and is truly a terrific healer.

Physical exercise: Working out the tension of anger through activity is important. If you chose an object on which to vent your anger, use pillows, bean bags, etc. but do not use pillows that you use everyday. Once you have vented your anger on the pillow you don't want to sleep on it - you will be literally sleeping on your anger.

Forgiveness: Contrary to what people believe forgiveness is an act that benefits the victim more than it does the perpetrator. When you are angry, you are the one feeling tense, uncomfortable, seething and obsessed. Letting go through forgiveness will enable you to free yourself of these unpleasant and disruptive feelings.

Imagery: There are various imagery exercises that help with your anger.

Anger Control Image

Imagine something that has happened to you that that you think is very unfair. It feels like a great injustice to you. You are feeling very angry. You are feeling very red inside. It feels as if your anger is a great ball of gas trapped inside you. There's a balloon near you. Pick it up and start blowing into it. As you do all that gas that is your anger is being exhaled from your body into the balloon. As you feel the balloon inflating you can feel yourself getting calmer. As the balloon inflates it gets bigger and redder. The balloon is now filled. Tie a string on the end of that red hot balloon. Take the balloon and go outside into your back yard. Now, you have that big red balloon on a string and you are standing outside your house. It's time to let go. You let go of the string. The balloon launches into the blue sky. Watch that balloon take off. Watch it going higher and higher up towards the sky, the red balloon going up into the deep blue sky. Watch it as it soars above the tree tops. Keep watching it as it gets smaller and smaller, going higher and higher by a flock of passing birds. You can still see it now, as it soars up into the deep blue sky. It is getting smaller and smaller. You can barely see it. It is just a dot now, fading , fading and now completely disappeared from view.

Frustration Control Image

You are feeling frustrated. Take your feelings of frustration. Get a suitcase and open it up. Put your feelings of frustration in the suitcase. Now close the suitcase Now you are going to take the suitcase into the attic. Pull down the attic stairs. Turn on the attic light Pick up the suitcase and climb the attic stairs. Put the suitcase down in a dark corner. Come down the stairs. Don't forget to turn out the light. Close the attic stairs. Well done! Now you can get on with your life. You can go and get the suitcase anytime you want - if you have to.

Sharing: Talking about your feelings with a sympathetic, empathic person is very valuable. The person could be a trained professional or a confidante whom you can trust. They do not need to be solving your problems - merely listening to them and allowing you to vent . If it is possible to take action to rectify your perceived injustice, so much the better but this should be in the interests of resolving conflict not merely getting revenge.

Using Anger Constructively.

Anger is a terrific motivational force and it can sometimes be harnessed to your advantage. I have known many people who have taken control of their life and their eating under the most trying circumstances, like abusive marriages, unsupportive family environments and personal setbacks. All of these people used their anger to motivate them and give them determination that they might not otherwise have.

If you are angry enough you can give up anything

Emptiness and Depression

It is part of the human experience to long for constant, unconditional love. Unfortunately, constant, unconditional love is not possible although we like to uphold this illusion. The closest we get to it is when we fall in love and experience the early stages of romantic love. Unfortunately, those moments are all to fleeting and we revert to the recognition, that when all said and done, we live this life alone, if not on our own. There are times when all of us come face to face with this aloneness and it can be experienced with a lot of sadness, worthlessness and emptiness. It is hardly surprising then, that people often try to fill this spiritual emptiness with physical fullness. These moments are often the setting for emotional, uncontrolled eating.

There is only one way to manage this feeling of emptiness. It is to put meaning in your life. Putting meaning in your life means having fulfilling relationships.

> **Five keys to fulfillment**
> Treat others as you would like to be treated
> Do not judge
> Listen carefully
> Be Mindful that Life is short
> Remember that your most important assets are your dignity, your humility and your love.

> **Physical fullness does not compensate for spiritual emptiness**

Depression

Depression is a word that means many different things to different people. There are many types of depression and many routes to it. Depression is not sadness, it is more a problem of reduced energy and lethargy.

While loss of appetite is a key symptom in the psychiatric diagnosis of depression, many people suffering from forms of depression tend to increase their food intake. Because depression is associated with lethargy, a depressed person often runs the risk of eating more, being far less active, and as a result, gaining a considerable amount of weight.

If you have any symptoms of depression, you owe it to yourself to seek help from a competent mental health professional. There are several effective anti-depressant medications and other treatment methods (like cognitive therapy) that can be really effective in reversing depression.There are things that you can do for yourself, depending on how much energy you have available.

Physical activity: You can jump start your energy system with even a modest activity program like the one outlined in this program. Increasing your physical activity may be the single biggest thing you can do for yourself.

Social activity: There is a terrific tendency to isolate yourself when depressed. This compounds the distorted thinking that accompanies depression and prevents you from getting important reality checks on your thinking, attitude and behavior. Force yourself into social situations - even if it is just for a few minutes at a time.

Sorrow grows in loneliness

10 Key Symptoms of Depression

Loss of energy	No enthusiasm in interests
Loss of sex drive	Poor sleeping
Change in eating habits	Tearfulness
Increased alcohol/ drug intake	Social isolation
Negative thinking	Low self-esteem

Tension
The three main ways of managing tension are:

Physical activity
Physical activity helps dissipate some of the extra energy created by tension and changes in body chemistry enhance relaxation. Any form of continuous movement, from vacuuming to strenuous exercise, is likely to help.

Mental relaxation
High levels of emotional arousal can be reduced through relaxation procedures, like the meditation exercises outlined earlier.

Distraction
Use your coping list to help get you involved in other activities, even if it's only for a short time.

Changing Distorted Thinking and Unrealistic Expectations

The ability to monitor and modify thinking habits is our greatest power. Here is an example of how thinking habits can influence a wellness or weight control program.

Let us suppose that it is the first day of your "program." You have done very well all day and are feeling very good about your effort and commitment. At the end of the day, you find yourself face-to face with your favorite, high fat, food. The chances are high that your first, automatic thought is something very similar to one of the ideas listed below:

> I've been good all day, I deserve it
> Just one piece won't matter
> I am going to blow it: I knew this wouldn't last
> I'll start again, tomorrow
> I'll start again, next Monday (even though today is Tuesday)
> I have got to have that
> I'll feel better if I eat it

The chances are high that this sort of thought will flash across your mind - and *that is okay.* If for decades, that's how you have reacted to your favorite food, it is unreasonable to expect that to change overnight, if at all.

The issue is not that you have this thought - the issue is how are you going to manage it.

Just because a thought flashes across your mind, does not make it true, valid, right or something you have to immediately act on. **YOU HAVE THE POWER TO CHALLENGE AUTOMATIC THOUGHTS AND CONTROL YOUR REACTIONS TO THEM.**

As you learned in the previous chapter, "mindfulness" is the ability to challenge automatic thoughts by subjecting them to a reality check. This technique applies to all aspects of life, not just eating. One definition of maturity: The ability to prevent destructive, automatic, habitual thoughts from adversely influencing your life.

Thinking Distortions of Bingers

Bingers and emotional eaters have some very specific thinking distortions about food, eating and themselves. These distortions need to be challenged and changed.

1. **Perfectionism** The binger typically sets themselves impossible standards. Setting high goals is not a problem in itself unless you are so inflexible that obstacles result in paralysis. Standards can be set so high that they prevent the person from even trying. Nobody is perfect and it is not possible to maintain a program perfectly. You do not have to be perfect. You only have to do enough of the right things, enough of the time, to make a difference.

Success depends on perseverance not perfectionism.

The single biggest characteristic that differentiates the successes from the failures on health and weight loss programs is that the *successes persevered and the failures did not.*

A perfectionist can easily be spotted. She will be the one who acts as if 1000 calories is bliss and 1001 calories is damnation. She will be the one who says she follows the programs she tries perfectly - for about four days and then gives up. She will be the one who will give up on a program after a "bad" weekend even though she has been very successful on it for three months. She is the one who will ignore all the progress she has made and focus on her inadequacies.

So my message to perfectionists everywhere who might be trying this program is:

Lighten Up!
⇒ Allow yourself a treat once in a while.
⇒ Do not be rigid about your caloric intake - be satisfied to fall within a range as suggested by this program
⇒ Remember you are going to have bad days - you are only human
⇒ Don't be discouraged - persevere
⇒ Give yourself credit for your progress

> The best way to scale down your weight is to lighten up your outlook

Anticipating the Worst
Many bingers/emotional eaters are first-class worriers. They see the pitfalls in everything and imagine the worst case scenarios so well that they experience their fears as realities. This only creates more anxiety. Almost all anxiety is anticipatory - it is fueled by imagining negative outcomes. This negative automatic thoughts need to be challenged. There are various ways to conduct such a reality check.

- Seek out and evaluate any evidence for your thoughts and assumptions
- How would you react if a friend told you the same thing?
- Talk to someone sympathetic
- Talk into a tape recorder
- Write your thoughts down
- How important is this in the context of your life generally?
- Will you remember this in six months time?
- Write down the opposite view

A good question to ask yourself:
Is this the way I *habitually* react in this situation, or is this unique to this particular occasion?

Ignoring the Positive
Because they set themselves fantastically high standards, bingers and emotional eaters are often blind to the progress they have made. This all-or-nothing thinking can be really destructive when considering a long-term, lifestyle change, which, by definition, is going to take time and occur relatively slowly and in stages.

It is important, therefore, to put the proper perspective on your progress.
- Do not necessarily compare yourself with where you hoped to be, but where you were six months ago.

- List any changes you have made

- Write down the best moments you have had.

The Love Affair with Food

Many people fall in love with food. When you fall in love, you project all the wonderful qualities you are desperately seeking onto your loved one. With people, this fantasy lasts a short time, because sooner or later reality will reveal that the knight in shining armor has armor that is in need of a thoroughly good polish, or does not really shine that much or worse still, is not even a knight. In short, we get disappointed because our lovers are human beings.

Food, however, does not seem to disappoint us. It generally makes us feel good, if only very fleetingly, and it doesn't answer back. As a result, food tends to be completely overvalued.

Food does answer back. The very same peanut butter sandwiches that give you temporary relief from boredom and frustration also:

> Fill you with guilt, and even shame and despair
> Add inches to your hips
> Clog up your arteries
> Ruin your self-esteem
> Force you into the next size up
> Make you feel out-of-control

Remember that the comfort you get from food is always short-lived. Satisfaction typically lasts as long as the food is in your mouth.

You need to get more realistic about the real value of foods that comfort you.

Cravings:

Here are some important things to remember about food cravings.

⇒ They are fleeting. They often pass quickly if you can resist your initial thought.

⇒ Craving is inevitable. Just because you have it, you don't have to give in to it.

97

⇒ Each time you successfully resist a craving you have made significant progress.

⇒ You will not die if you do not satisfy a craving.

⇒ The more prepared you are, the better off you will be.

Step Five

Temptation: Winning the Tug-of-War

Oscar Wilde once said, "I can resist anything but temptation." Temptation is the downfall of many people on a weight control program. Many of my clients have said they felt as if they were in a constant tug-of-war, with willpower on the one side and a demonic, evil, tempting force on the other. In this chapter I will tell you about self-control and how to develop it, especially in reference to temptation and craving. I will tell you why temptation occurs and what you can do to control it. The exercises that accompany this section include some essential retraining exercises involving actual behavioral assignments and some imagery work that will be really helpful in your battle against temptation.

What is self-control and where does it come from? If you have self-control in one area of your life does it generalize to others? These are difficult questions with no easy answers. But I do know that self-control is not something that you either have or do not have. It can be developed and in this section of the _7 Steps To Wellness_ program I will tell you how to improve your self-control.

When we are talking about self-control in a weight management program like this one we are really talking about managing temptation and craving.

Managing Temptation and Craving

Temptation is a normal and natural phenomena. It happens to all of us. If you make no attempt to resist temptation, like people not concerned about their diet, then temptation is not an issue. If, however, you are constantly fighting temptation, it's significance grows. **Like anything else in life, the more you resist a force the more you empower it.** Now, that doesn't mean I am suggesting you simply give in to every temptation - far from it. But what I am saying is that the power of the temptation lies in your approach to it rather than any intrinsic energy it has on its own. Temptation does not have to be the setting for panic. The more confident you become of your temptation management, the less power it will have over you.

Having a craving for a food does not mean you are unmotivated, lazy, shameful or evil. Temptations can occur as a function of many things; fatigue, exposure to your favorite foods, habitual thoughts about food, certain environments and settings. Temptation is normal. Being tempted is not the problem - it is how you manage the temptation that is the issue. Sure, you would like to go through life never being tempted by food again - that would be the easy way. Unfortunately, it is completely unrealistic. Temptation will not go away. You can take steps to minimize it and can you learn to manage it but it will not disappear. Unfortunately, too many people assume that temptation is somehow going to magically disappear the moment they decide to embark on a weight management program and are disappointed in themselves when it does not.

The Origins of Craving
Why does temptation occur? Sometimes temptation can occur because of physical reasons. You may be fatigued at a low energy point of the day and your body will start demanding more food. Energy is a very important concept that is often overlooked as an explanation for behavior. Energy fluctuates during the course of the day. When energy declines, desire for food increases. When does energy drop to low levels? Around the middle of the afternoon and late at night, times typically associated with craving and bingeing. Eating small frequent, healthy snacks and keeping physically active are the best ways of managing energy slumps.

Another physical cause of temptation is blood-glucose level. Falling blood sugar levels stimulate an increased desire for food, often experienced as a temptation or craving. Blood-glucose levels fluctuate for a number of physical reasons. Moderate to large sugar intake can create swings in blood glucose level, as can hormonal changes, especially around menstruation. Both of these situations can be eased by eating small frequent meals, rather than large infrequent ones.

There are also more subtle influences on the development of temptation. Once again, we return to the two great principles that govern all human behavior, association and repetition. Consider the following example.

Let us suppose that each evening at about ten o'clock, as you wind down before retiring, you take a candy bar into the bedroom and eat it while relaxing in front of the television. This is part of your relaxation routine. Let us suppose that you started doing this when you were going through a stressful period and you found that this habit helped you relax.

The more you repeat this behavior the more it is encoded into your nervous system. The more you repeat it, the more eating candy bars is associated with relaxation, ten o'clock at night, your bedroom and watching television. The more it is associated with those things, the more power those things have to elicit temptation and a desire for the candy bar.

Now, as it approaches ten o'clock and you enter you room, your body goes Aha! time for a candy bar. Your stomach starts to produce gastric secretions in anticipation of your candy bar. This makes you feel more hungry - what I call *pseudo hunger* - a conditioned eating response. You would not have felt hunger if you were not in this situation. This environment triggers the pseudohunger /AHA response. In fact, AHA stands for a scientific term - A Anticipatory, H Homeostatic, A Adjustments. That is more of a mouthful than a fistful of your favorite peanuts so let me explain.

Body Memory
Homeostasis is the process by which your body keeps its systems on an even keel. It is a system of checks and balances. If your blood-sugar increases, insulin is produced to bring it back down. If you go into a dark room, your pupils dilate to allow more light in. If you go into bright sunlight they constrict to minimize the amount of light. These basic homeostatic processes happen all the time within your physical system and are a marvel of creation. Each time this happens your body is making a homeostatic adjustment. If your body finds itself in a situation that is characteristically and habitually associated with eating, it is adaptive for it to anticipate this and make an *anticipatory homeostatic adjustment*. Your body learns with repetition that eating takes place in that situation and anticipates it. Thus, as you enter the bedroom, your body recognizes that this is an eating place and time and starts to prepare for that incoming candy bar. Depending on how well practiced this particular habit is, your body might just make a few gastric secretions, or

it might even produce some insulin in anticipation of a rise in blood-sugar. These secretions will make you feel - hungry. This is one of the reasons why in this situation you will find it difficult to break this habit - if you try not to eat the candy bar you will still feel the pull of your *pseudo hunger*.

Now knowing about this mechanism and changing your behavior are two quite different things. Understanding this mechanism will help you realize that fighting temptation is not just about being lazy or unmotivated. There is a real physiological mechanism at work. This knowledge is not sufficient on its own to enable you to change, however. In trying to change any behavior, retraining is more important than knowledge and in the exercises that accompany this section I will guide you through assignments that will indeed help you break these habits. Be assured, however, that these habits can be changed. If your body has learned this association, then it stands to reason that it can unlearn it, too. With enough repetition of retiring at ten o'clock and not eating the candy bar, this association can be unhooked, your body will learn not to associate candy bars and this environment, your pseudo-hunger/aha response will disappear and your temptation and craving will fade. This sounds easier said than done. How do you break the cycle to begin with?

Developing Self Control
Many years ago when I was a postgraduate student at the university of London, my colleagues and I investigated just this problem working with alcoholics. We wanted to see whether practicing abstinence during repeated exposure to a tempting situation, in this case alcohol, would reduce the experience of temptation and craving. In an experiment that probably could not be conducted today, we had alcoholics who had given their informed consent, in a controlled environment, sit in front of their favorite alcoholic beverages while attempting to resist drinking. (If you have a drinking problem, please do not try this at home! This was an experiment conducted in a very controlled environment under special circumstances) What we found was that the experience of resisting in this very difficult situation did reduce the experience of craving and improve the subjects' ability to resist temptation. This work formed part of my Ph.D, in which I also found that subjects' ability to resist temptation was enhanced if they had initial practice in doing the whole thing in their imagination first. Technically this approach is called cue exposure with response prevention - being exposed to temptation but not
102

indulging - and there are many treatment centers around the world that now use this technique. Whatever name is given to the technique what you are really doing is developing self-control.

It is hardly surprising that imaginal practice is helpful. There is much evidence that suggests that mental practice really enhances performance. There is also some evidence that imaginal practice is powerful at a symbolic level, too - influencing the primitive brain in a way that simple knowledge does not. So practicing successfully resisting temptation in your mind, without the real exposure to tempting foods, is the first step in managing difficult temptation situations. I am going to guide you through the development of your self-control, one step at a time. As you master one step, we will move to the next and so on until you have really developed your self-confidence and control.

Once you are able to imagine yourself successfully dealing with temptation, you will be guided through assignments in which you come face-to-face with real-life tempting foods. We will start with foods that are not necessarily your all-time favorites and build up to the point where you can resist your favorite foods more effectively.

In asking you to confront your favorite foods and temptations in this way, I am not asking you to do something that does not happen already - you are confronted with temptation almost daily. I am trying to get you to confront temptation in a controlled way, on your terms and with some specific tools.

One of my former colleagues called this technique of confronting temptation rather than avoiding it, brinkmanship. In this case you are pushing the limits of your ability to resist food to the brink.

This is a self-paced procedure. If you think that you are getting into situations that you cannot manage - do not do it. You are the best judge of what you can manage so do not go beyond what you feel is manageable. Moreover, if you really believe that you can eliminate certain foods completely from your life and you do not want to mess with them, do not bother working with them in these exercises. If, however, you want to be able to eat many of your favorite foods in moderation, or if you feel that you want to control foods rather than have them control you, then these exercises will help you.

Several important points follow from seeing craving and temptation in this way. Temptation is a natural and normal part of life and you can learn to manage it. More importantly, the best opportunity to develop self-control comes precisely when temptation is at its highest. Life teaches us that most growth occurs at the time of maximum difficulty. **Being faced with temptation is an opportunity to develop your self control.**

Some years ago a client announced that immediately following her participation in my weight management program she was going on a week's cruise. On the face of it this did not seem terribly good planning. Using the self-control principles I have outlined here, she was able to manage the temptations implicit in a cruise and called following her trip to proudly announce that she had lost three pounds while on board. More importantly, however, she said that the experience of successfully dealing with a difficult situation really increased her level of confidence in being able to manage temptation. "If I can be successful on a cruise, I can be successful anywhere," was her comment. Your perception of your ability to manage a situation, what in psychology is called your self-efficacy, is directly related to you performance.

On another occasion, a client was learning about these self-control exercises while staying on a boat owned by one of his friends. One night, several unannounced guests arrived and proceeded to party on the boat. Not only was this an intrusion for my client but it also brought him face to face with his all time favorite temptation - honey roasted peanuts. Using the self-control techniques he was able to master the temptation, a feat that heretofore had not been possible. "It just would not have occurred to me that I could resist," was his comment.

Like these two people, you too can learn to resist temptation. There will be occasions when you will want to indulge yourself - and that's perfectly okay, too. Once you have learned to develop self-control, it is likely you will be able to eat some of your favorite foods in moderation. Your approach can be one in which you control the food, not the other way around. Rather than feeling defeated and out -of-control you can approach temptation with more confidence.

Temptation can be very transient and fleeting. The chapter, "Coping: Putting Out Fires" contains strategies for delaying your response to temptation and helping you define coping mechanisms that work . If you see temptation as a normal, natural phenomenon, you are much more likely to be able to manage it. The more you develop self-control the less threatening and powerful temptation will become.

Well, so much for the behavioral training of self-control, what about the psychological side of managing temptation.? What can be learned from the mindfulness exercises that could help in the management of temptation.?

The Psychology of Temptation

People overvalue certain foods. As already outlined in the chapter on bingeing, many people have a love affair with certain foods. You will hear some people actually say, that they "love" chocolate ice cream, or they "adore" cheesecake. Now if you have read enough pop psychology you will know about love. You will know that the early stages of romantic love are an illusion - a trick to bond people together. You will know that in the early stages of romantic love we project onto our new found partner all sorts of wonderful characteristics that we want them to have. This dreamy, illusory state of ignorance is very intoxicating, especially since our partner is similarly projecting on to us all sorts of wonderful qualities that we may, but probably do not, possess. After a while this illusion fades leaving us to face a different sort of reality.

Because they are imperfect, human beings will inevitably disappoint the person that has too high expectations of them. Food, on the other hand, does not talk back, is not moody and does not get headaches. We can thus continue to project onto food many wonderful qualities and never feel that it is going to disappoint us. We can continue to cling on to the notion that the chocolate mousse is really going to make us feel better and that the Baked Alaska is going to energize us, despite the fact that all the evidence is that you feel good for the few seconds that you are tasting the food but thereafter you feel either nothing or downright bad.

The mindfulness exercises included with this program helped you check the reality of your thoughts about food. And to break some of your fantasies, and in particular the emotional links you have with your favorite foods, I have included as part of the self-control exercises that accompany this section the chore of throwing away some of your favorite food. (Down the disposal, where it can not be possibly retrieved!) I am not suggesting this procedure as an everyday tactic but as an exercise in breaking strong emotional ties that you may have with certain foods.

Fighting Talk

All this is very well and good but what are you going to say to yourself in a temptation situation. Let us suppose you have been doing this program for a few days and are managing well: You are starting to walk on a regular basis and feel that you are making progress in getting it all together. Then, one evening at a social event you come face-to-face with your all time favorite food. What is the first thing that is going to flash through your mind?

If you are anything like the majority of people to whom I have posed this question in the past, and you are honest, you will admit that the first thing that will flash through your mind in this situation is something very similar to "I've got to eat that!"

This will be followed, at the speed of thought, with some rationalization why you should indeed allow yourself to eat it. Variations on this theme include, "I've been good all day, I deserve it," "I'll start again tomorrow," "I'll start again on Monday," (a particularly liberal commitment if today happens to be Tuesday) or "One piece won't matter." Whether one piece will really matter depends largely on your perception of what it means to eat just one piece. If indeed you are able to eat one piece and eating it does not bother you in any way and it does not trigger further temptation, then one piece really does not matter. If, however, you think that eating one piece means you have violated your program and that you are now off track and are feeling despondent and defeated, having just one piece will matter very much.

It is perfectly okay, natural and normal for the first automatic thought to flash through your consciousness to be a desire to eat. You have probably been thinking that way for many years, even decades, so it is quite unreasonable to expect that to change just because you make a commitment to watch your weight. In fact, that initial thought might never change - and that's okay, too. It's not having the thought that's important it's what you do with it once you have it. Managing the
106

thought is the key. So what is really important is not your first thought but the second, third and fourth thoughts that you use to challenge the idea that this food has absolutely to be eaten.

Of course, the front of the buffet table may not be the best place to stand and have a heated debate with yourself about the merits of your eating and besides it may be too late - you may have already eaten it! In the event that the temptation is overpowering, arguing with yourself is not the best tactic - just beat it out of there as quickly as possible. For more strategies in this situation you are referred to the next chapter "Coping: Putting Out Fires"

So here you are with a desire to eat that cheesecake - how are you going to talk yourself out of it? What thoughts can be mustered to help you win this particular tug-of-war with the devil.

Well there is nothing like a little reality to throw cold water on the best of fantasies. *The best way of countering tempting thoughts about food is to consider what eating the food will really mean to you.*

Yes, eating that cheesecake may make you feel good for the few seconds in your mouth but what about later? What about later when you are feeling depressed, out-of control and generally not feeling very good about yourself? What about later when you can not get into your favorite outfit or see your reflection in the mirror? What about later when you have heartache, heartburn or a heart attack? What about later?

Thinking about later is the trick. The short term consequences have far greater influence on our behavior than intermediate or long term ones. **The real challenge in life is making the long term consequences influential on your present behavior.**

When you think about the long term consequences in this context you will see that whether they are concerns about your appearance, mental state, mood or health they represent your motivation. In fact, they tie right back into the exercises you did earlier in the motivation module. If you have developed strong motivational images, if you can stay mindful of your worst fears and best hopes, if you can keep those motivational messages and images in front of you they will be an enormous help in your management of temptation.

In summary, the secret to the successful management of temptation lies in controlling the habitual physical and mental impulses you have when you first encounter the temptation. The specific behavioral exercises designed to help your self-control will give you more control and, if nothing else, will help you to buy time. You can buy time to talk yourself out of the temptation by focusing on the reality of the long-term consequences. The motivation exercises, along with the reminders of your real motivation, should help give you effective tools in doing this.

The self-control exercises can also help you buy time to escape the situation by distracting yourself or physically removing yourself from the immediate danger.

Developing Self-Control
There are five phases in the development of self-control. As you have just read, it is necessary for you to:

1. Identify your temptations and tempting situations
2. Develop and practice thoughts that will counter the immediate urge to eat
3. Imagine yourself successfully resisting temptations
4. Put yourself in situations where you actually successfully confront these temptations
5. Learn to throw some of your favorite food away

Identifying temptations and tempting situations
Identify those foods that you consider, on their own, constitute a strong temptation.

1..
....

2..
....

3..
....

4..
....

5...
....

Identify those situations that you consider, on their own, constitute a strong temptation.

(Examples: Middle of the afternoon, alone in my kitchen)
1...
....
2...
....
3...
....
4...
....
5...
....

Now you have identified temptations it's time to learn how to manage them.

Developing Counter Thoughts

Imagine you are in a highly tempting situation, Your favorite food is in front of you. You really want to eat it. What could you say to yourself to help you avoid eating?

(Tip: refer to your motivational exercises for some ideas.
Examples:
I don't have to eat this
This is going to make me depressed
This will only feel good for a few seconds)

Now it is your turn
1...
....
2...
....
3...
....
4...
....

Resisting Temptation in Imagination
I am now going to guide you through four situations in which you overcome temptation or inertia.

When doing these exercises find a comfortable place where you will not be disturbed. Take some water with you and have it readily available.

In this first scenario you will imagine yourself sitting in front of the television in the evening and feeling tempted by ice-cream. *If Ice-cream is not a temptation for you substitute some other food that is.*

Imagine you're at home - it's about nine in the evening and you're watching television. (If you never do this substitute some other activity like reading). You're a little tired but enjoying some relaxation time. Suddenly you get the thought that it would be nice to have some ice-cream. You know you have some in the freezer and the more you think about it the more idea grows that it would be good to have some ice-cream. Imagine going into the kitchen. There's nobody else around. You walk over to where that ice-cream is kept and take the container out of the freezer. You can feel the ice crystals from the bottom of the container as you carry it to a counter top or table. Open the container - it looks good. You can almost taste it. You get a dish and start to spoon the ice-cream out of the container. You can see it, almost taste it. As you are spooning the ice-cream into the dish it occurs to you that while the ice-cream might taste good for a few seconds you will feel out of control and frustrated. That while the ice-cream might taste good for a few seconds you will feel that you have negated all of your effort and that in eating the ice-cream you will consume the same number of calories in a few seconds that it will take you an hour of exercise to burn. Imagine picking up the container and putting it back in the freezer. Walk back over to the dish of ice-cream. Take the ice-cream and through it down the garbage disposal. You can hear the whirr of the disposal as the ice cream washes away. As the ice-cream disappears down the disposal you feel in control.

How did you do? It may have been difficult for you to imagine throwing the food away. Don't worry if it was - with practice you will
110

find it easier to be able to see yourself throwing the food away. Remember throwing away food is not mean to be an everyday tactic but a way of *breaking your emotional ties with food.*

Did you salivate during this exercise? If you did, it shows how powerful these food-body associations can be. If you feel hungry, drink some water. Keep practicing this important visualization.

Let us try another one. In this scenario you are going to imagine being at home, bored in the middle of the afternoon and tempted by some junk food. *If junk food is not a temptation for you substitute some other food that is.*

Imagine that you at home, alone, in the middle of the day. You are having a tough time getting started on anything - you're bored and distracted. That high fat food that you have in the refrigerator starts to seem very appealing. Imagine going over to the refrigerator and taking the food out of it. See yourself putting the food on a table or counter top. The food is right there in front of you now ready to eat. Look at it - you can smell it, almost taste it. It looks really good you - you really want to eat it. You are about to eat it when you see yourself on the scales, upset and frustrated at having gained weight. Although the food will taste good for a few seconds you don't what to get derailed. Imagine yourself taking the food and throwing it away. As you watch the food disappear down the waste disposal you feel good about being in control. You feel good that you control the food not the other way round.

How did you do with this one? If you felt frustrated and angry throwing the food away - keep practicing. Take some water.

The next situation involves overcoming your resistance to taking a morning walk.

Imagine that it's that time of the morning when you are scheduled to take your morning exercise. Imagine that you really do not want to do it. You don't have any energy and don't want to go. But a voice from somewhere inside you tells you to go - even for a few minutes. Taking a walk might give you some energy. Imagine putting on your walking shoes and heading out the door.

Try this last one.

Imagine that it's lunch time. You're feeling hungry but you're also in a rush. You decide to head to your favorite fast food restaurant. See yourself driving into the drive-thru lane and stopping by the order board. You can see your favorite fast food meal. You can almost taste the fries. Imagine ordering a salad instead.

Practice these self-control exercises at least once. This will take about ten minutes. Once you have practiced the self-control exercises you can adapt your own special situations and practice successfully resisting them.

Now that you have learned the principle of the self control imagery you can adapt your visualizations accordingly. In your imagination, practice successfully resisting situations that are particular problems for you.

<u>**Confronting Real Temptation**</u>
Whenever you find yourself in a tempting situation, remember *this is the best opportunity to develop self-control Use the counter-temptation thoughts and imagery to help you cope.*

Deliberately seek out tempting situations to practice your self-control. If you are doing this, remember:

- Only expose yourself to those situations that you think you have good chance of resisting
- You can limit your exposure to a few seconds if necessary
- Don't practice this exercise when you are hungry
- Make sure you have water, juice or diet soda available
- Plan to have something to do immediately after the exercise

Examples:
Bakery - Try this exercise if baked goods are a problem for you.

<u>Goal: To be around baked goods but not indulge.</u>

<u>Step 1</u>: Go into your favorite bakery. Look at the foods that tempt you, inhale the smell, then walk out.

<u>Step 2</u>: The same as above but stay a little longer - a minute or two rather than a few seconds.

<u>Step 3</u>: Go into the bakery, sit and have just a cup of coffee but do not indulge in the baked goods.

You could repeat the same exercise for ice-cream/yogurt stores, cookie and candy stores.

Remember this is an exercise in developing self-control. If you do not feel that you could be successful at a particular exercise do not try it. **People learn more by trial and success rather than trial and error.**

<u>Throwing Away Your Favorite Food</u>

The purpose of this exercise is to break some of the emotional ties you have with food, treat food as a disposable commodity and develop some mastery over your favorite food. <u>Do not eat for ninety minutes after doing this exercise.</u> Ways of making this task easier include:

- Do it with somebody else present, particularly someone trying the same exercise.
- Don't do the exercise when you are hungry
- Have something planned immediately after you do the exercise
- Don't have other tempting food available.
- Make sure you throw the food down the disposal.

<u>What about the starving children in...?</u>

Many people have guilt about wasting food. This typically comes from past experiences where food meant fulfillment, satisfaction and love. This is precisely why this exercise is so powerful and necessary - you need to break that association. You should never eat because you feel you have to please someone. **Eat for hunger, eat for pleasure but do not eat for obligation.**

If you are really concerned about starving children, don't buy junk food and send the money you have thus saved to a reputable charitable organization that really helps with world hunger. I know for certain, that your consumption of that cookie, ice-cream, yogurt etc., will not help one starving person.

Now a short test to see if you've been paying attention.

What does AHA stand for?

What happened to the woman on the cruise?[13]

---

[13]   *Answers: Anticipatory Homeostatic Adjustments; She lost three pounds*

Step Six

Coping: Putting Out Fires

Throughout this program I have been urging you to remember that your theme should be 'Progress not Perfection'. There will inevitably be times when your motivation ebbs, when life ruins your best plans and when things aren't going the way you want. If Albert Ellis , the famous rational-emotive therapist were here, he would be saying "Who ever told you to expect that life would go smoothly?"

No, life does not go smoothly and as if the ups and downs of life are not enough to contend with, we know that there are going to be situations that present special challenges to you and your ability to stay with the program. Being successful on a program like this one involves accepting several realities. You need to be flexible in your goals and what you expect to accomplish at any given time. You need to adapt to the particular situations that you face and you need contingency plans to counter predictable and unpredictable high risk situations.

Many, if not all, of the situations that can create problems for you, however, are <u>predictable</u>. Eating out at restaurants, holidays, vacations, dinner parties, special events, travel are all very predictable and yet few people plan effectively for them. Effective management of high risks is not difficult - it requires planning and practice. It is well worth it - **prevention is better than panic.**

As outlined in the self-management chapter, awareness is the key. You need to know what situations pose a threat to you. Using your weekly meeting with yourself to anticipate upcoming risks will help you prepare for problems. As well as <u>specific, unique</u> situations, there are a cluster of situations that most people find difficult. In this chapter I will show you how to make effective contingency plans. In addition, there are certain behaviors that are universally useful and I will help you define which of these work best for you. Here are the golden rules of risk management.

Managing Hunger

The fist point is simple but fundamental - never get really hungry. This may sound obvious but is often overlooked. If you get really hungry the chances of making good food choices become virtually nonexistent. Many people believe that skipping meals will help them lose weight, but this simply is not the case. If you skip meals you eventually get hungry. At this point you feel virtuous as well as hungry and then justify excessive eating on the grounds that you've been good all day. This makes no sense, is not healthy and is a recipe for failure. It is absolutely essential to eat something at each meal time to prevent this from happening. Even if that something is a piece of fruit or some cereal or just a piece of toast - eat something at meal times.

There are some occasions when it seems like you do not have a chance to eat for hours at a time. I have heard many people say "I just don't have time to eat." This does not make sense. It does not take very long to eat a piece of fruit or a sandwich - maybe a few minutes. It probably takes less time to eat a healthy snack than it does to go to the bathroom and you do not hear many people say "I have not had time to go to the restroom today." The key here is to ensure that you have a piece of fruit or a sandwich or a healthy snack easily available. Planning this in advance should not tax the average brain. It is a good practice to carry at least a piece of fruit and a healthy snack bar with you in the event of emergencies. Keep it in the car, in the office, in your pocket book - and please remember to change it once in a while if you have not needed to use it.

Eating regularly, especially small meals and snacks, will help keep your blood-glucose level stable. When blood sugar starts to bounce all over the place - as it does if you eat larger, infrequent meals - hunger and craving levels increase dramatically. I know several people who have been very successful in controlling their weight by switching to a regime of small, frequent (about every two hours) healthy snacks.

The "never go hungry" rule also applies to the timing of your evening meal. Do not wait until your spouse is ready to eat - by that time you might be ready to eat the furniture. A light snack or a salad can moderate your hunger for a couple of hours and make your appetite more manageable. One of my clients calculated that an apple held off his hunger for about an hour and a half and with practice you will learn how different snacks moderate your hunger levels. This is not an invitation, however, to have two dinners.

Focus

Maintaining focus is the second rule of prevention. Use the Personal Healthscope to keep track of your behaviors. When things are not going well it's easy to lose focus. Always try, however, to maintain awareness by tracking your behavior regardless of how well you are doing.

A contingency plan is the most urgent requirement when you find yourself in that rut. Good contingency plans typically involve activities like sharing, exercise or immersing yourself in something that interests you. The exercises in this section show how to plan and implement good contingency plans.

The third golden rule involves exercise. Unless you are physically unable to move, *do some physical exercise* - even if it's just for five minutes. Maintaining a reasonable exercise routine will inoculate you against disaster. If you keep exercising you are far less likely to regain weight, unless your eating is wildly out of control.

Research suggests that about twenty-five per cent of people get derailed from their exercise program by injuries. Do not exercise if you are in pain or have an injury that has not been attended to by a qualified professional. Seek appropriate medical advice for injuries. Rest is often all that is needed. You are far better getting the injury treated and being sidelined for a week than ignoring it and being sidelined for three months. If you do have a minor injury you need to exercise sensible judgment. A broken toe nail is not a reason for abandoning your exercise program. Alternative exercises are useful both as a change of pace and as a way of minimizing strain on the same parts of your body. If formal exercise as such is not possible, consider ways to be more active generally. Do not exercise if you have pain and certainly do not ignore an injury.

Maintaining a Routine

It takes a lot of effort to establish a routine so you don't want to abandon it too quickly. Once you have stopped a routine it is downright difficult to get it restarted. It is a common myth that it takes three weeks to change a habit. This particular folk wisdom is misleading. It might take three weeks of doing a behavior for it to become something you expect to do but the real question is how *robust* or enduring is the habit? The question is not how long does it take to start doing a behavior on a regular basis but at what point is that behavior so established in your repertoire that even if you stop it for a short while you will go back to doing it. It might take as short as three weeks to start doing a behavior on a regular basis, but it takes far longer than that, probably at least a year, before that behavior becomes an enduring habit.

Apart from your regular exercise routine, you can also find ways of increasing your general activity during the day. The obvious suggestions here include walking rather than relying so much on mechanical devices like cars, elevators and escalators. There are other ways of simply increasing your activity. My suggestion for phone walking (outlined in the exercise guide) is a good example of how to burn off a few extra calories during the course of everyday activities. If you have a portable phone simply walk (in ever decreasing circles if you have to) while on the phone. If you spend a total of an hour a day on the phone the number of calories will add up and make a significant contribution to your weight control effort.

Damage Control
Implementing damage control is the fourth golden rule. Too many people consider their weight program an all-or-nothing proposition. If they cannot follow their plan exactly they do not follow one at all. This is the biggest difference between people who are successful and those who are not. I have seen many people who have lost a lot of weight - many of them in excess of a hundred pounds - and every one of them said that they had bad days but they just kept going the best they could.

Once you have got off track it is difficult to overcome your inertia and get started again. Try to keep as much as possible of your program going.

Even if you are having difficulties, minimizing fats and keeping as physically active as possible should be your goal. The idea of someone eating a cheeseburger and fries and then opting for a diet rather than a regular soda may seem a little absurd but the fact is the diet soda is a better choice than the regular one, no matter what else you are putting in your mouth. Every calorie and fat gram saved adds up. Remember, most weight is cumulative - it goes on slowly over a period of time as a result of many small decisions made throughout the day.

Golden Rule number five is **be realistic**. There will be times when it is unrealistic to expect to implement your program fully. This is particularly true when people are trying to get back on track after they have slipped for a while. In this situation, guilt drives people to gear themselves up for a great motivational push and they set unrealistic plans.

For example, one of my clients had slipped from the program. She had done very well in losing about thirty pounds but then had stopped because of a number of stresses in her life and had started to regain weight. Once she survived her life crisis she was ready to tackle the plan with renewed vigor and enthusiasm. Despite the fact that she had been bingeing and overeating considerably for a while, she planned to immediately cut back to less than a thousand calories a day. Despite the fact that she had not exercised in a couple of months she planned to walk three miles every day.

Well, it is tough to go from eating pretty much anything you want to restricting in one fell swoop. She did not eat less than a thousand calories on the first day back on her program. She ate about fifteen hundred - quite an achievement in my view but not in hers. She was not satisfied so the next day she redoubled her efforts and ate about twelve hundred calories. This was ideal in my view but a failure in hers. Although she was able to walk for four miles on the first day, she was somewhat sore and barely walked at all the second day. Again, a good start in my view but a failure in her eyes.

My recommendation to her was to concentrate on cutting back the fats and sugar and not be too concerned with overall volume of food. I also suggested that she plan to start walking just ten minutes a day. If she had set these goals form the beginning, her transition from being off track to in control would have been much smoother and less stressful. Once she accepted the need for realistic goals she was soon back on her program.

Setting realistic limits for yourself - especially when you are restarting your program - is crucial. You have to consider where you have come from if you are going to plot the best course to where you want to go.

With these golden rules in mind, let's consider certain typical problematic situations and plan how to manage them effectively.

Dining Out

First consider situations in which food is a focal point of a social gathering. Plan to minimize temptation by taking as many precautions as possible and have effective contingency plans in the likely event that temptation will occur. Guidelines to managing in specific restaurants are provided in the Dining Out guide

Ways of minimizing temptation include choosing an appropriate restaurant and going with people who will support rather than sabotage you. If you have friends who will be good role models for you, so much the better. It so much easier to exercise healthy choices if the people around you are doing the same.

Mental practice improves real life performance so mentally rehearsing the whole scenario, from ordering to exercising control, is useful. Remind yourself of your motivational images so that you can stay focused on your goals. At the restaurant, order first, having decided your order in advance.

Portion size can be a major downfall. Control portions by asking for a specific size, splitting entrees or making your own meal out of available appetizers.

Do not go hungry and help offset excessive hunger by having some water and /or a salad before the main meal arrives. Watch out for alcohol. Willpower dissolves in alcohol, so once you have had a glass of wine (or its equivalent) be careful. Note that after three glasses of wine, alcohol facilitates fat storage.

Sauces and salad dressing often have a high fat content. Be very careful in your selections and always order these on the side. Which reminds me of story that highlights an important point in all of this risk management advice.

A woman approached me after one of my seminars and told me she had been very successful after following some of my advice. She proceeded to tell me that my words had made a profound impact on her

120

and she had been able to lose a substantial amount of weight. As she was saying this I was wondering what gem of wisdom I had given that had made such positive impact. Perhaps it was the work I had encouraged her to do on developing self-control? Perhaps she had spent weeks and weeks practicing the self-control assignments and finally had achieved it for the first time in her life? Perhaps I had helped her mine her motivation and now armed with this weapon she had been able fight off temptation? Perhaps I had been able to help her stop bingeing and regain control of that area of her life? Which of these nuggets had the desired effect?

As I was considering these options, I have to admit to feeling a little satisfied that fifteen years of training and twenty years of experience had borne fruit in this particular case. As I was considering which of these brilliant therapeutic strategies had the greatest impact she said, "Yes, what helped me last year was when you said, take the salad dressing with you." After I picked my self up from the floor and talked to her more, I realized that what she was saying was that even the most simple strategies can be very helpful. In her case, for whatever reason, taking the light salad dressing with her to restaurants symbolized her ability to control the situation. It was the perception of control that was so empowering to her. Obvious tips can be helpful. Remember, **common sense is not always common practice.**

Variations on the restaurant contingencies apply to other food-focused social situations. Similar contingencies apply to cocktail parties, for example. Do not go hungry. Minimize your exposure by arriving late and leaving early. Do not position yourself by, on or under the food table. Focus on the conversation. Have a soft drink in your hand at all times. Decide to eat nothing, easier if you have dinner plans in your immediate future. This is not complicated. It is not brain surgery. (On one occasion, I ventured to suggest to my audience that this whole process was not brain surgery only to discover that indeed there was a neurosurgeon sitting in the audience. The next time I gave the seminar I changed my metaphor and said, "This is not rocket science." As luck would have it there was a NASA engineer in the audience.)

Dinner Parties

Dinner parties present different challenges. If you know the hostess well enough you might be able to gauge the likely fare and you might even feel comfortable enough bringing a dish or two of your own, a tactic of many vegetarians. If none of these options are available, do the best you can. It is not the end of the world if you make the decision to ease up a little on your program for any particular occasion.

There is no need to feel self-conscious at a dinner party. Most of the women and many of the men at such an event are also concerned about their diet. Very few , if any, will be watching exactly what you eat.

Although most people will readily accept medical reasons for almost any behavior, I suggest you do not fabricate some mysterious illness to justify your restraint. I know of one woman who felt that she had to justify her refusal of dessert on the fabricated grounds that she was taking medication that precluded her eating the chocolate mousse. Unfortunately, she neglected to find out that the guest to her right was a pharmacist who immediately inquired as to the nature of this medication. She had to endure an awkward moment when there really was no need to put herself in this position. A firm 'no thank you' is all that is required (if you do indeed decide not to indulge.) You do not need to justify your behavior to anyone. Neither do you need to be militant. Pointing to the chocolate mousse and declaring that "Anyone who has any of that is going to have a coronary on the spot - I'll call 911 now, to get them prepared," is an unnecessary comment. The best way to influence others is by example not by running commentary.

Holidays

Holidays present special challenges, combining as they do exposure to the double trouble of both food and family. Setting realistic goals is once again the key. Thanksgiving is probably not the best time to aim for a thousand calories a day. There is absolutely nothing wrong with going for maintenance rather than weight loss - increasing your calories, without going crazy. Be aware of what you are eating, still consider low fat or fat free alternatives, and keep up some sort of exercise. Similar rules apply to vacations, where, in theory at least, there is more time and opportunity to be active. You should consider your opportunities for activity when planning your vacation, or at the very least when making your accommodation arrangements.

In the exercises that accompany this section, I want you to identify the situations in your life that present special problems and to devise some contingency plans to handle them effectively. Remember, the more plans you have, the more likely it is that one or two of them will really work.

Surviving Temptation
The situations in which temptation and craving occur are predictable, so planning really helps. Temptation can be very fleeting. In fact, if you can survive the first few seconds of your exposure to a tempting food your chance of resisting it altogether increases substantially. Do not panic. Your goal should be to *survive the first minute* and work from there.

An airline pilot once told me how he had been trained to respond to an emergency. If the alarms sounded in his cockpit his first response was - do nothing. He was trained not to react reflexively - that could be disastrous. He was trained, when the alarm went off, to sit on his hands and analyze the crisis and then respond in a considered way. He cited one European airline disaster that was directly attributable to an inexperienced co-pilot reacting too quickly. This co-pilot had apparently acted reflexively when an engine blew and switched the engine off. The only problem was that in his haste he switched off the one remaining good engine and the plane crashed on to a highway. You do not want to crash and burn Take your time. The food is not likely to disappear. It is not the last time you are going to see this food. You can always get it if you want it. Do not panic.

Let me share with you some simple strategies that will help you not to panic and that will help you buy some time.

Your first response might be to immediately get a glass of water (or diet soda.) This gives you something to do on your initial exposure to temptation, will put something in your hand and in your mouth, will fill you up and buy some precious time. Leaving the environment is often an option. If your co-workers are in the habit of producing cookies and doughnuts in the middle of the morning you could always absent yourself - take a walk or use the time to make calls.

Distracting yourself by getting involved in other activities is important and in the exercises that follow I will get you to consider what options are open to you. You do not have to distract yourself for hours at a time - surviving a difficult few minutes is all that is necessary.

The strategies I have just mentioned concern the beginning of eating but two useful tactics concern the *continuation* of eating and may stop you eating too much.

The first involves delaying your decision to eat more. Once you have eaten the intended amount, delay eating anything more for about twenty minutes. That is not to say that after twenty minutes you can not go and get more to eat, but delay further eating for twenty minutes. This is effective and here's why. It takes about twenty minutes after you have ingested food for you to start feeling the effects of that food as far as fullness is concerned. You could be stuffing yourself silly but there is going to be a twenty minute lag before you feel the effects of satiety. These twenty minutes are therefore a dangerous period as far further eating is concerned. This is one reason why slow eating is encouraged. If you wait the twenty minutes before having the dessert, for example, you will find it a lot easier to resist.

The situation is worse than I have described. Not only does it take twenty minutes for the feeling of satiety to set in, eating primes further eating. In the twenty minutes after you have started eating, you are more likely to want to eat. So delay further eating. Leave the table and get away from food if you have to. When you leave the table, get involved in an activity unrelated to food. If you go back into the kitchen, you are going to be around food again, and then we know what's going to happen to the leftovers.

A tactic that has helped many of my clients in this situation started out as a tip to help smokers quit. This simply involves going to the bathroom and brushing your teeth. Not only is this good dental practice but it will make you mouth feel clean, change the tastes in your mouth that may be contributing to your temptation and will get you away from food. Moreover, if you have associated the bathroom or teeth cleaning with some of your motivational messages this will help, too.

I hope that you have understood that managing difficult situations is itself not difficult. Spending a few minutes considering what strategies work for you can literally save you a lifetime of misery. So I strongly encourage you to do the simple exercises that accompany this section. It could make a world of difference.

Improving Coping Skills
In all areas of life, preparation and training pay big dividends. If you are going to be successful in maintaining weight you have to identify the situations that are the greatest potential risks and deal with them before they defeat you.

A study conducted some years ago that investigated the strategies used by people who were successful in changing their behavior revealed the following information. People who were successful:

1. Maintained "cognitive vigilance." "Cognitive vigilance" is just an academic's way of saying, "Keeping focus." People who were successful kept aware of their goals and their behavior.

2. Used a range of coping strategies to prepare for and deal with potentially risky situations.

In short, thousands of taxpayers dollars were used to reveal that people who were successful kept their focus and planned for difficult situations.

Planning & Scanning
Here are the typical problem situations.
Restaurants
Vacations
Holidays
Cocktail parties
Travel
Dinner parties
Cooking
Guests
Special events

Restaurants

In the Temptation Management section of this program you have already practiced visualizing successfully managing the temptations implicit in a restaurant situation. The Dining Out Guide gives you helpful hints on how to manage eating in restaurants. In this section, I want you to consider what are the biggest problems that you face in a restaurant and how you are going to deal with them.

10 Problems With Restaurants And What To Do About Them

I never go to the restaurants that would be most helpful to me
Be more assertive
Go alone or find someone who wants to go the same restaurant
Almost all restaurants have healthier, if not healthy, alternatives

The people I go out to eat with sabotage my program
Choose supportive people to eat with
Take an enforcer
Ignore them and use your anger to meet your goals

I am always starving by the time I get to eat
Insist on going earlier
Eat something prior to going
Drink water and order a green salad as soon as you sit down

I eat too much bread and butter before the meal
Ask for the bread to be removed
Eat the bread but not the butter
Have a salad (with no or low fat dressing) instead

I get too easily tempted by what I see others ordering
Order first
Don't even look at the menu
Order (Decide) ahead of time

The portions I eat are too big
Specify small portions
Split entrees
Make a meal out of the Appetizers

Once I have a glass of wine or two my willpower dissolves

Don't drink
Used fruit juices instead of wine, non-alcoholic beers
Used mixed drinks and alternate with soft drinks or water

I never know what is good to order
Ask how food is prepared: avoid fried, battered and pastry
Ask for dressings and sauces on the side
Consult the Oracle(HealthScope)

I am a sucker for dessert
Have fruit or low-fat dessert
Have a Capuccino
Beat it to the restroom and stay there while others are eating dessert

I do great at the restaurant but eat up a storm when I get home
Eat more healthy food
Bypass the kitchen and go straight to bed
Don't have anything at home to eat

General Tips:
Don't go hungry
Drink plenty of water
Wear tight clothing
Brush your teeth immediately you finish (in the restroom, not at the table)
Take fat free dressing with you
Don't linger, especially with food on the table
Visualize being successful beforehand
Useful phrase at a restaurant
"I am allergic to fat and I will die if I get too much of it."

Write down ten things that you can do that will help you in a restaurant.

1..
2..
3..
4..
5..
6..

7. ....

8. ....

9. ....

10. ....

Visualizations

You are now going to work on imagining coping successfully with some high risk situations. To get the maximum benefit from these exercises you need to find a comfortable place where you will not be disturbed. So turn down the ringer on the telephones and tell anyone else in the house you are not to be disturbed.

In the first scene in this section, I am going to guide you through a restaurant situation.

Restaurant

I want you to imagine you are going into a restaurant. You are going with some of your friends. See yourself entering the restaurant. Now you are being led to the table by the hostess. You are all sitting down. The hostess hands menus to your party and you are all now looking at the menu. As your friends look at the menu they start talking about ordering high fat foods with creamy sauces, fries and butter. Although this sounds tempting, you know that if you eat them you will feel out-of-control, fat and miserable. Think about how much it means to you to be in control, looking good and feeling healthy. The server comes back to the table. You quickly place your order for a healthy alternative It feels good to be in control.

Dinner party

Imagine that you are at a dinner party .You have just finished the main course and have managed to eat a healthy meal. Coffee is being served. The hostess comes up to you and asks whether you would like a piece of the dessert that is her specialty. It looks very good. You can hear other people raving about it. You can smell it, almost taste the texture of the food in your mouth. You realize, however, that it will taste good for a few seconds but after that you will feel as if you have got off track and negated all the effort you have made until now. You look your hostess in the eye and say, "It looks great, perhaps I will have some a little later." As your hostess smiles and walks away you feel very pleased and relieved.

128

Office

Imagine you are at the office. It's in the middle of the afternoon. The day is beginning to drag a little. One of your co-workers comes by with a big plate of doughnuts and cookies. Look at those doughnuts. They are your favorites. You can smell them, almost taste them. But as you look at them a little more closely you can see the fat oozing out of them and you can almost feel the greasiness. You can see the large grease spot on a napkin where one of these doughnuts has been sitting. You can feel your waistline expanding as the fat cells fill up with the fat from the doughnut. You look at your colleague and say, "I don't really want one, but thanks for the offer."

Now that you have learned the principle of the self control imagery you can adapt your visualizations accordingly. Now, in your imagination, you can practice successfully resisting situations that are particular problems for you.

Holidays & Vacations

A reasonable goal on a holiday or vacation is to *maintain rather than lose weight*. Most people would be very happy to return from a vacation not having gained weight.

When I am on vacation I feel as if I can eat anything I want

You can eat anything you want, you're just going to pay the price if you overindulge
You can still eat a good volume of food as long as its relatively low-fat
Occasional indulgences are fine but don't abandon your overall commitment to your health and weight goals.

When I am on vacation I get out of my usual routine

Try to keep as much of the routine going as possible
Use the HealthScope on a daily basis
Do some exercise

When I am on vacation I don't have access to exercise equipment

Plan your accommodation near or at a facility that has equipment
Plan to compensate by taking small equipment with your
Improvise

129

When it is a holiday I feel as if I can eat anything I want
Stay aware- monitor your fats and calories
Increase volume but not fats - choose low-fat or no-fat alternatives
Watch out for alcohol which will dissolve your willpower

When it's a holiday my family always has a large meal
You can still be vigilant and choose healthier alternatives
Have the meal, enjoy it but plan for it - and don't try to compensate by missing meals, just get back on track

When it's a holiday I sedate myself with food to cope with relatives
Minimize your exposure to your relatives
Keep exercising - even when they are talking to you
Really try to listen to what they are saying

<u>Cocktail parties and dinner parties</u>
When I'm at a cocktail party I eat lots of small hors d'oevres
Refrain from eating anything
Stay away from the food
Keep count

When I'm at a cocktail party I drink too much
Mix drinks with juice, water or mixers
Stay with soft drinks
Abstain

Total abstinence is easier than perfect moderation - St. Augustine[14]

When I'm at a cocktail party I use food to overcome the boredom
Remember that food does not make the talk any more interesting
Arrive late, leave early
Try to make the talk less boring

---

[14] He was referring to sex but a similar principle applies to food and alcohol in these situations

Dinner Parties
When I'm at a dinner party I find it hard to resist the host's hospitality
Accept what you want to accept and graciously refuse the rest
Being gracious is not the same as being intimidated
Sometimes avoiding "hospitality" is the best way of avoiding the hospital

When I'm at a dinner party I like to eat dinner
Eat what you want and enjoy it
Keep vigilant
Once the meal is finished try to keep away from any lingering food

What are your other high risk situations?
What are your special high risk situations? List them below.

1..
....
2..
....
3..
....
4..
....
5..
....

The Master Coping List

To deal with these situations you need coping strategies. Take a few minutes to make a master coping list - a list of all the things you could possibly do to deal with your identified risks. When making your master coping list you need to bear in mind the following principles.

Be Specific. For example, do not just put down "exercise", list all the exercise you could do in that situation. Do not just put down "call friends"- itemize, line by line, all the friends you could call and write down their phone numbers.

Think of places you could escape to. Leaving a tempting situation is sometimes the best policy. If you do leave a situation where are you going? Friends' houses, the Mall, the movies, the library, the park, the gym and the church are all possibilities.

Consider others who can help you. Sharing and communication are often the best ways of coping. In each situation, who could help you the most?

Consider activities and situations that are incompatible with eating. Typically the more active you are, the less likely you are to eat. There are also places where eating is less likely (e.g. the library) and some where it is more likely (e.g the mall).

Your master coping list should look something like this.

Situation
Bored in the middle of the afternoon at home
Coping list
Take a fifteen minute walk
Swim twenty laps
Call Karen 123 4567
Call Anne   123 4568
Clear out attic
Go to the movies
Go to the library
Do some yardwork
Catch up on correspondence

Situation: **Lunchtime at the office**
Coping List
Take a healthy lunch with me
Take a fifteen minute walk
Do resistance exercise with free weights
Meet friend for healthy lunch
Catch up on calls
Call Lisa 123 4570
Do fifteen minutes relaxation/meditation
Practice visualizations

Make a coping list for each of your high risk situations. Each list should contain at least ten things you could do when faced with that situation.

The longer you can resist a temptation the more likely you will be successful. Your goal is to delay an impulsive response and survive the first few seconds of your initial exposure to temptation.

First Response ideas
Drink a diet soda/water
Brush your teeth
Take ten deep breaths
Call someone
Go for a walk

Now a short test to see if you have been paying attention.

1. People accurately estimate how much they eaten in the past twenty-four hours. True or False?

2. Self-monitoring is not important in order to successfully manage your weight? True or False?[15]

---

[15] Answers: False. People typically underestimate calorie consumption by at least 50%. False. Self-Monitoring and awareness are crucial.

Step Seven

Support: Erecting Fences

Changing behavior is difficult enough to do without sabotage. Unfortunately, changing your lifestyle is sometimes enthusiastically opposed by important people in your life. Having the support of others is helpful but not necessary. Early in my career when I was young graduate, a colleague and I approached a nutritional company with a proposal to research the role of social support in successful weight loss. As experienced as we thought we were in the subject of weight loss we were completely green in business. As we were waiting in the lobby to make our presentation we met a commercial photographer. In the course of the conversation he told us his daily rates of pay. Realizing we had substantially undercut ourselves in our proposal, we hurriedly rewrote our estimates and ending up getting the contract at double our initial proposal.

The small study which we ultimately completed, researched women attempting a weight loss program in supportive and non-supportive environments. We found that some women in non-supportive family situations turned their anger into a positive force - it made them more determined and eventually successful. Some women who seemed to be well-supported at home could not use it effectively, while others thought they were being supported but were actually being undermined.

Regardless of the outcome of our small study, it is ideal to have the support of significant people in your life.

Social pressure is a huge influence on our behavior. We live in a society where individualism is the dominant philosophy. Although the notion that anyone can do anything if they just try hard enough is empowering, it does substantially underestimate the role of other people in our environment.

To give you an idea of the immense power of other people's views and social pressure consider these two classic psychology experiments from the 1950's and 60's.

Social Influences
The first is a classic experiment conducted by a social psychologist called Asch. In his experiment, he introduced subjects into a room where a group was already assembled. The experimenter then asked the group members some simple questions about a some drawings. One of these questions concerned two lines A and B, in which B was obviously shorter than A. When the group members were asked which of the lines was shorter everyone else in the room said A (probably because they had been instructed to do so by the experimenter). Suppose you are in this situation. Everyone has endorsed a particular answer, now it's your turn. B looks shorter than A but everyone else has said A is shorter - which do you choose? Under these circumstances a substantial number of people go along with the group, despite the fact that it is obviously the wrong answer. Why?

Subjects who endorsed the wrong answer might have had the following thoughts. "I'm sure the answer is B, but everyone else said A so I must have misheard the instruction." Or they might have thought " I know the answer is A, all these people are crazy, let me get out of here as quickly as possible and to heck with the experiment." Or they might have actually *seen* A as shorter. Other research suggests that perception can indeed be altered by suggestion. In any event, the experiment shows that our behavior, if not our perception, can be changed by what other people say and do.

When I was a young adolescent I grew up in London right around the corner from Wembley stadium, the site of big soccer matches. Every other year, England played Scotland there in a sort of tribal warfare. Thousands of Scots would descend on London for the match. I always managed to get into the game and one year I did so only to find myself surrounded by thirty thousand somewhat inebriated and fanatic Scotsmen. I was fifteen at the time and although I was wanting England to win when I got to the stadium, when I found myself surrounded my thought processes changed. Suddenly it seemed quite acceptable if Scotland were to win. After all, look at all these people who had made the long trek south. (Actually Scotland scored two goals in the last five minutes and did win and I lived to tell the tale). Have you ever gone to dinner with the best of intentions only to get derailed by dinner partners who have different health goals? Resolve melts and rationalizations pop into your mind as they encourage you to indulge.

Suggestibility

It is clear that some people are much more influenceable than others. Suggestibility is a function of experience, personality and age. We are more subject to influence when we are younger. In the Asch experiment mentioned above, for example, college freshmen were more likely to be influenced by the group than seniors. All of us have our limits, however, and we are influenced by social pressure much of the time. Consider this famous experiment conducted by psychologist Stanley Milgram at Yale during the 1960's. If you had been a subject in this experiment you would have been led into the experimental room and shown a piece of equipment designed to deliver electric shocks to a person sitting in another room. You would have been told that your role in this experiment is to ask that person in the next room some questions. If they give the wrong answer you have to give them a jolt of electricity. If that was not bad enough, each time they got a question wrong, you have to increase the voltage of the shock. At this point you are shown the shock delivering equipment and you can see a meter that stretches across a continuum that goes from mild shock to extremely dangerous. You start the experiment and much to your dismay (or maybe delight) the person in the other room is not very smart. Before long you are having to deliver increasingly painful electric shocks. They are getting so painful, that the person in the other room is crying out in pain, asking for the experiment to be discontinued. If you are like most of the subjects in this experiment you will turn to the experimenter and ask him what to do. He will quietly tell you that the experiment must continue. Now, what do you do? Well, 62% of the subjects continue to give increasingly painful electric shocks, all the way up to the maximum level on the shock box meter. Interestingly enough, when subjects were debriefed the most common reaction by far was relief, not anger as you might expect.

This experiment was considered a landmark in understanding the tremendous influence of expectations, social role and other people. Changing your behavior is likely to be threatening to many people, especially those close to you, so you had better be prepared for dealing with their reaction. You have just encountered the first rule of stress: Whenever there is change there is stress.

The Reactions of Others

The first rule in dealing with others is to recognize that each of us has our own ax to grind. Each of us wants as much control as possible and will manipulate like crazy to get it. We all see life through our own neurotic lenses. **There is no need for you to be deflected from your goal because of other people's neuroses.**

You will get an array of reactions from other people as you proceed with your program and wellness efforts.

Some people will be truly pleased at your progress and be supportive and encouraging. Some, however, will have a more negative response.

There will be some, who will, quite frankly, be jealous. These people may such things as, "I think you're getting too thin" after you have lost just a couple of pounds. Or they will comment on the difficulty of keeping weight off. They might make other disparaging comments.

Many women are unhappy with their weight. Nearly everyone wants to be even a few pounds thinner and many women struggle most of the waking lives with the thought of reducing their weight. It is hardly surprising that some of them will be irritated when they see others being successful. The jealous remarks should be simply ignored. Consider such comments as a sign of flattery. If they are jealous they must think you are being successful.

Not that jealousy will come only from women. The man in your life might also be jealous that you are getting your health act together while he is not. Weight per se is less important to the man than his perception of his fitness. Women talk about losing weight, men merely talk about "getting in shape." Many men talk about getting *back* in shape when it is not entirely obvious they were in shape to begin with.

Gender differences in body weight perception are important. Genetics contributes significantly to these differences. Throughout most of the animal kingdom, successful females, i.e. those high up in the pecking order, are slender while those lower down the order are fat. In the animal kingdom however, the situation is reversed for males - the higher up the pecking order the male is the heavier he is, while the low-order males are thinner.

Other Sabotaging Strategies

Sabotage can be expressed in ways other than jealousy. Friends and family member sometimes make it easier for you to deviate from your program. The common term for this form of sabotage is *enabling*. I think *disabling* is a more appropriate term. Such disabling is often done with the best of conscious intentions. There's the husband who rewards his wife for losing weight by buying her a box of chocolates. Or the mother-in-law who bakes your favorite high-fat pie even though you have been telling her for the past month about your new health program. How do you handle such situations?

It is easy in these situations to feel that tact is the better part of valor and simply give in. There will be times when that is an appropriate tactic. After all, there is absolutely nothing wrong with having a modest piece of pie, especially if you feel that you can manage eating it without losing control. A piece of pie, or even a chocolate or two, will not hurt you unless you perceive eating it to mean that have lost control. There will be times, however, when you really do not want to eat the pie - as much as you don't want to disappoint your mother in-law. Alternatives in this situation include taking a piece and slipping it to the dog, or dropping it into the vase or even out of the window. As you do this you say something like, "That was really sweet and thoughtful of you, and even though I am on a special program and really working hard to watch what I eat, I will take a small piece because you went to all of this trouble just for me." **Remember, the medium is the message. It is not as much what you say as how you say it.**

If, however, these disablers are part of your daily life, you have to take more permanent action.. You need to explain, rationally and calmly, reasons for your new behavior. Explain why their support is so important. It is easy in this situation to tell disablers what not to do. It is far better to take a more positive approach. It is tempting to blast your husband for being inconsiderate, selfish and sabotaging when he disables your program but this is unlikely to have the desired effect. This highlights a few key principles about communication that you need to implement if you are going to get what you want.

How you say something is as important as what you say. The non-verbal aspect of your communication is going to determine the listener's attitude before you have even delivered your message. If you storm into

138

a room, your listener is already on the defensive and preparing to reject your message even before hearing exactly what it is.

Assume that most people are going to be resistant to your message. Your goal as an effective communicator is to overcome the listener's resistance. Attacking, criticizing and berating your listener is not likely to breakdown their resistance, it's going to dramatically increase it. Which is why Dale Carnegie, in his classic and insightful book, "How to Win Friends and Influence People", says that you can never win an argument. Getting mad, has a role to play. Venting anger may make you feel better and it might have a certain dramatic effect, but its overall value as a communication tool is not high.

You need to break down your listener's defense not build it. Presenting messages in a form that is acceptable to the listener will reduce resistance. For example, to the disabling husband, who brings home chocolates and cakes when you are obviously trying to avoid such foods you might *want* to say something like:

"You're a sabotaging, insensitive slob who has absolutely no interest in my well-being. I am appalled by your selfishness, thoughtlessness and lack of concern, not to mention respect."

But what would be more effective is:

"Honey, I know you are really trying to support me on my program, and you are encouraged when I do well. What would be really helpful to me is, when you want to show your enthusiasm for my efforts, as a treat you bring me some of those fat free chewy rewards - I am really hooked on those and they are good for me, too."

You have not alienated him, you have got him to identify with your efforts, you have labeled him as supportive, you told him how he can support you and - you have even got him to do some of the grocery shopping too!

Not only have you wrapped up your message in a way that is acceptable to him you have also taken the first step in effective communication. You have got him to identify with you. You have labeled him as supportive and have begun to get him to relate to what

139

you are doing. Never, never interpret other people's motives back to them. This is a job for the skilled psychotherapist - do not try this at home! Do not try this for two reasons. One, you are going to be wrong a lot of the time. Two, even if you are right, the last thing any of us wants is to be given interpretations about our behavior. It is one of the surest ways of escalating an argument, polarizing your listener and increasing his resistance.

Control Freaks

All of your communication skills will be tested to the maximum if you have to deal with control freaks. These are people who will tell you that your approach is wrong, that the menu plan needs changing and that you are not doing the right exercises. They will tell you all of this despite being a little overweight themselves and leading a lifestyle that could hardly be described as healthy. Even if they are the epitome of fitness, it does not give them the right to impose what worked for them on you. The word here is *impose*. Recognize that what works for one person does not necessarily work for another.

It may be possible, if the controller is not a constant in your life, to give them the impression that you have heeded their advice, even if you have not. Perhaps they have suggested (control freaks do not really suggest they tell, if not demand) to you some tactic that you are already using. You can thank them and tell them that you will adapt their suggestion.

In the last analysis, however, if you are living with a control freak, this particular battle will have to be fought. Remember, you have more power in this situation than you think. **People only have power over you if you have given it to them.** Abide by the basic principles of effective communication described above. Do not interpret their behavior. Talk about *your* feelings, thoughts and behaviors not theirs. Get the listener to identify with you and your efforts. Show how the other person can be supportive.

A study conducted at Purdue University some years ago by Dr. Randy Black identified four types of support. Informational support is simple education. For example, the number of calories in a particular dish. The second source of support is encouragement, the proverbial "pat on the back" for achieving a goal. Facilitative support occurs when a
140

person performs an action likely to elicit healthy behavior in the program participant. For example, rather than slump on the sofa immediately after dinner and exercise the remote, your spouse says, "Let's go for a walk." After you have fainted, you can pick yourself up and accept the offer. The fourth and most important support occurs when another person provides balance and a reality check when your thinking gets distorted. An example of this would be your spouse reminding you of your overall level of progress on a day when you were discouraged.

Getting Support
If you have all of the above mentioned supports in your life, particularly the last two, you are very lucky. But if you do not, *ask* for them. Show your spouse and other family members and friends how they can help you. If you ask for support and get it really show your appreciation, even if it was not done in exactly the way you would like. Don't forget that this is often new territory for your spouse and family so they need support and encouragement, too. This point was brought home to me some years ago when I was counseling a couple who were having difficulties in their marriage. Poor communication was their main problem. Several sessions were spent exploring the husband's apparent inability to express his feelings. During our fourth session, he triumphantly if somewhat clumsily, expressed a genuine emotion. Rather than acknowledge the effort he had made in expressing himself, his wife immediately criticized the content. In response to this criticism the man he stood bolt upright, said "That's why I never I say what I feel," and promptly stormed out of my office never to be seen again. Those around you are learning new behavior patterns too. Treat them as you want to be treated. All of your relationships are special but the marital one holds some specific pitfalls in the area of lifestyle change.

Is Marital Neutrality Possible?
Many women participating in my groups wished their husbands would not get involved in their programs.. They wished they would be left to get on with their program by themselves. This is often an unrealistic wish. Many overweight women are not happy with their bodies. This dissatisfaction affects their comfort with intimacy, their sex life and their mood. In this situation, the husband has obviously got an emotional investment in his wife's weight and her comfort with her body. A man in this situation, watching his wife eating cream pies will see her devouring his sexuality as well as a large number of calories. Neutrality
141

is not possible. Obviously the relationship between sexuality and eating and weight is complex and will not be covered comprehensively here. Women do need to understand, however, that their husbands do have an emotional investment in their weight and eating, just as much as a wife would have an investment in her husband's excessive drinking. **The secret to effectively dealing with these issues, like everything else in marriage, is team work.**

The Negative Thinker

Joining the saboteur, the disabler and the control freak in the rogues gallery of obstructive individuals, is the negative thinker. The negative person says things like; "You look like you've lost a few pounds but I bet you won't keep them off. Everyone knows it's impossible to lose weight." Or " If you keep exercising so much you're going to get injured." Try to resist the temptation of giving these people an instant frontal lobotomy. These people can really inspire you. If you are struggling to get up and out to do your walk, just think of these nihilists gloating over your failure. Anger is a great motivator. **If you are angry enough, you can give up anything.**

Other than that, simply ignore these people, or humor them. If they say "I'll bet you'll be off this program in two months," you reply, "Do you really think I can keep it going that long?"

You Have the Power

In all of these situations there is something fundamental to remember. You have the power. Any power others have you have given them and you can get it back at any time. In the written exercises that follow you will be asked to identify the people in your life that fall into various categories of saboteur. During one of my seminars, we were doing this exercise when one of the participants made an insightful remark. "There's one person who appears in each of these categories," she volunteered. Of course, I was curious to find out who this was. "It's me," she said. In that simple exchange she said a lot about dealing with others. Dealing with others begins with dealing with yourself. You may have fears that you are not doing it right, that your motivation is going to fade, that there is a better way of doing it and that you are going to fail. If you do have these negative thoughts it is easy for someone else to hook those anxieties and reinforce them.

You can only do your best. Do not get bogged down in too much thought. Avoid paralysis by analysis. This is your life, your mind and your body. As Rabbi Susya says, "God will not ask me why I was not Moses. He will ask me why I was not Susya."

Responsibility

No-one else has responsibility for your life and no-one else is going to take care of it. This does not mean to say that you should not listen carefully and consider what other people are saying to you. Even a good idea expressed in an off putting manner is still a good idea. If an acquaintance sees you eating a candy bar and says to you, " You know, that's not the best choice, if you wanted a snack, this fat-free bar is much better," you might be tempted to react by saying something like, "Who asked you?" storm off and eat three more candy bars. Okay, so she did not say it as tactfully as she might, but the *content* of the idea I still valid.

Which brings me to the last point about dealing with others. If at all possible, surround yourself with people who are supportive. As you learned at the beginning of this chapter, other people are powerful influences on our lives and we want to make that power work in our favor. When going out to eat for example, try wherever possible, to choose your companions appropriately. People who are going to encourage you to substantially deviate from your plan are not helpful and the less you are around them the better.

Finally, when people are nosy enough to ask you how much weight you have lost, you have several alternatives. You can tell then the truth, refuse to answer them (just because somebody asks you a question you do not have to reply), tell them that it is not about weight but it is about how you feel and you are feeling great. You will feel great if you see yourself making the effort and taking control. **Reclaiming your personal power will make you feel terrific.**

Getting the Support You Need

In the exercises that follow, you will consider the people who influence you for better or worse. When completing these exercises, remember that the same people can be both positive and negative influences.

Who in your life is supportive of your efforts?

Use the grids below to identify the people in your life who are supportive and unsupportive.

(Example:

Name	Role	How do they support you?
Fred	*Husband*	*Walks with me*
Patrice	*Instructor*	*Encourages me, a great example)*

Now it is your turn.

Name	Role	How do they support you?

....

....

....

List other people in your life who could support you and what sort of support would you like from them?

(Example:

Name	Role	How could they support you?
Franny	*Friend*	*Acknowledge my effort*
Susan	*Supervisor*	*Allow me to take short walking breaks*

Now it is your turn.

Name	Role	How do they support you?

....

....

How could you get the support you want from these people?

(Example:

Name	Role	How could you get their support
Franny	*Friend*	*Talk to her, reinforce her when supports*
Susan	*Supervisor*	*Explain my program to her)*

Now it is your turn

Name	Role	How could you get their support?
....
....
....

List the people in your life who sabotage you and how they do this?

(Example:

Name	*Role*	*How do they sabotage you?*
Fred	*Husband*	*Buys me cookies, does not want me to lose weight*
Me	*Self*	*Too pessimistic)*

Now it is your turn.

Name	Role	How do they sabotage you?
....
....
....

How are you going to deal with saboteurs?

(Example:

Name	*Undermining behavior*	*Your new response*
Fred	*Buying me cookies*	*Throwing them away*
Fred	*Doesn't want me to lose weight*	*Ignore sabotaging talk*
Me	*Too pessimistic*	*Lighten up, Practice Mindfulness*

Now it is your turn.

Name	Undermining behavior	Your new response
....
....
....

How are you going to reinforce supportive behavior?

Here are some ideas of how you might reinforce the behavior you want.

- Say Thank you

- Express appreciation

- Buy a small gift

- Be reinforcing in return

- Communicate honestly

Now it is your turn.

....

....

And now a short test to see whether you have been paying attention.

Name the four types of support?

What percentage of the subjects gave the maximum level of shock in the Milgram experiment conducted at Yale?[16]

---

[16] Answers: information, encouragement, facilitation, balance; 62%

Nutrition

Sensible Food For A Sensible Weight

Diet and nutrition play a crucial role in wellness. Following a diet that is low in fat, especially saturated fat, includes essential vitamins and minerals and is moderate in sugar, caffeine, sodium is a necessity for maximum wellness and weight control.

In keeping with my philosophy of making things as simple as possible for you, however, I have devised this weight control system so that all you need to do is select from the recipes that have been provided by our dietitian, Colleen Wracker. These follow a sensible low-fat nutritional plan as outlined above and even allow for a snack. You do not need to be a nutrition expert to eat a sensible diet. If you do want to know more, however, Colleen and I have included a very basic description of the fundamentals of good nutrition so that you can understand the principles of this system.

There are many good books and articles available on the subject of sensible nutrition. We particularly recommend The Wellness Encyclopedia of Food and Nutrition from The University of California at Berkeley.

Fat Reduction

The single biggest component of a healthy diet is reducing the amount of fat. Although a certain amount of fat is necessary, we tend to eat too much of it. The current average American diet is about 34% fat. We could eliminate 75% of our current fat intake and still meet our fat needs! Excess fat in our diet contributes to heart disease, cancer and diabetes, three leading causes of death.

The technical name for fats is lipids. They come solid or in liquid form in the form of oils. All are insoluble in water. There are two main types of fat, depending on their chemical structure.

> **The more fat reduction**
> **The less liposuction**

The two main types of fat are:

Saturated fat:

Saturated fat is what many people consider "bad" fat. This is because saturated fat tends to increase the production of low-density lipoproteins (LDL) or "bad" cholesterol, a process which is implicated in heart disease. Saturated fats are not essential to health.

Saturated fats:

- Are typically solid at room temperature.

- Come mainly from animal sources. (Coconut and Palm oil are the exception in that they are saturated fats that come from vegetable sources)

  7% of your daily intake of calories should come from saturated fats.*

  This is the 7% solution!

> **Just be content**
> **With seven per cent**

This means your saturated fat intake should be:

no more than   8 grams on a 1000 calorie/day diet

no more than 12 grams on a 1500 calorie/day diet

no more than 16 grams on a 2000 calorie/day diet

Unsaturated fats

Unsaturated fats have one (monounsaturated) or more than one (polyunsaturated) double bonds in their molecular structure. Unsaturated fats are essential for good health. They are important in hormone production and in the health of cell membranes.

Unsaturated fats have other qualities:

- They are liquid at room temperature

- They go rancid quickly

- Plants and fish are the main source

There are two types of unsaturated fats:
    Monounsaturated (e.g. olive, canola and peanut oil)
    Polyunsaturated   (e.g. corn, sunflower and sesame oil)

It is preferable to chose monounsaturated fats rather than polyunsaturated fats wherever possible

Our Recommendation:

<u>**No more than 15% of your daily intake of calories should be taken in the form of unsaturated fat***</u>

A percent of fifteen **Will keep you lean**

This means that your unsaturated fat intake should not exceed the following:

      17 grams on a 1000 calorie/day diet
      25 grams on a 1500 calorie/day diet
      33 grams on a 2000 calorie/day diet

Percentage of calories from fat	
Cream cheese Most cheese and cheese spreads Eggs Regular ground beef Peanuts Pork (loin) Oil packed tuna & salmon Tongue	50% or more
Beef (Lean ground, Porterhouse, T-bone, Round, Rump) Chicken (roasted, flesh and skin) Lamb (shoulder, rib) Pork (fish and cured ham, shoulder) Salmon (red sockeye, canned) Whole milk	40% - 50%
Beef (sirloin, arm, flank) Chicken (dark meat, roasted flesh) Lamb (Leg, Loin) Pork (heart, kidney) Turkey (flesh and skin, dark meat)	30% - 40%
Beef (Heel of round, Pot roast) Chicken (no skin) Fish (Bass, Oysters, Pink salmon) Liver	20% - 30%
Bread Fruit Low fat cottage cheese Fish (Cod, haddock, water-packed tuna, halibut, sole) Most cereals (other than granola) Most shellfish Most vegetables Skimmed milk	under 20%

Get a good book that contains fat content of foods, including fast food and ethnic foods.

WARNING! It is convenient to express the recommended fat intake in terms of overall percentage of calories. This works providing you are eating no more than about 2000 calories a day. As your caloric intake increases, however, the percentage of calories from fat should decrease.

For example, 25% of a 2000 caloric diet is 500 calories, about 55 fat grams. But 25% of a 3000 calorie diet is 750 calories, or 83 fat grams. An intake of 83 fat grams is not consistent with a healthy diet. It is recommended that your intake of fat not exceed 60 grams daily.

Calculating fat grams

There are 9 calories per fat gram, regardless of whether it is a saturated or unsaturated fat.(This compares with 4 calories per gram of protein or carbohydrate).

To calculate the number of calories of fat eaten, multiply the number of fat grams by 9. (Now you finally have a use for the 9 times table you learnt all those years ago. Or else turn on your calculator)

If you have a product that has 10 fat grams it has 10 x 9 − 90 calories

If you have a product that has 10 fat grams and has a total of 100 calories it is 90% fat. (It has 100 calories and 90 of them are from fat, 90/100 = 90%)

If you have a product that has 10 fat grams and a total of 450 calories it is 20% fat. (It has 90 fat calories, 90/450 =20%)

Another way to calculate fat is to compare total fat grams to total calories. To make it simple, look for the foods that have about 20% of their calories from fat. This is approximately the same as 2 grams of fat per 100 calories or 4 grams of fat per 200 calories.

Fat Grams

Calculate the following:

If you have a product that has 5 fat grams and a total of 100 calories, what is the percentage of fat?

If you have a product that has 6 fat grams and a total of 200 calories, what is the percentage of fat?

Answers: 45%, 27%

Reading labels

Labels typically contain the important nutrition information but be careful of some common pitfalls.

Nutrition Facts

Serving Size

Servings per Container

Note serving size: It's often smaller than you think!

Check Servings per Container. Calculate how many calories, fat grams etc., there are in the **entire container!** Don't assume a serving is "one" serving, no matter how small it may be

Amount per serving

Calories   Calories from Fat

% Daily Value*

Total Fat

Pay attention to fat grams, **not the % daily value**

 Saturated Fat

Cholesterol

Sodium

Total Carbohydrate

Dietary Fiber

Sugars

Protein

Vitamin A

Vitamin C

*Per cent daily values are based on a 2000 calorie a day diet

Note that the calories probably are more than your goal !

Low-Fat Alternatives

There are now many low-fat alternatives on the market. These are generally an acceptable way of enjoying the flavors of your favorite foods while minimizing your fat intake. If you're not concerned about weight loss, these are very acceptable. If you are concerned about weight loss then remember that overall calorie intake (**even non-fat calories**) *do count.*

Be careful! We believe that the fat free alternatives are actually contributing to more food intake by some people. If you eat a lot of food, even if it is fat free, you will not lose weight and may well gain it.

When considering various low-fat alternatives pay close attention to the sodium and sugar content. These can be high when the ideal intake of sugar and sodium is moderate.

A low fat dessert **Is one that won't hurt**

Cholesterol

Research over the last two decades has shown conclusively that cholesterol is a major factor in coronary heart disease. Excess cholesterol leads to plaque which in turn, blocks arteries.

Our body naturally creates all the cholesterol we need, but because it is also in our diet, exclusively in animal products, we risk ending up with too much of it. Eating sensibly has been shown to be the single biggest factor in reducing cholesterol. Nutrition can help in two ways.

By limiting the intake of cholesterol, we can minimize the chances of excessive build-up. Cholesterol is found mostly in foods that are high in saturated fat. For example, 3 ounces of chicken liver has 540 mgs of cholesterol, but 3 ounces of skinned white meat chicken has only 77 milligrams. A large egg has 212 mgs but 3 ounces of fresh fish has 42 mgs.

Consume no more than 150 - 200 milligrams cholesterol daily

Cholesterol is carried between the liver and the cells in your body by lipoproteins. High Density Lipoproteins (HDL) are efficient carriers of cholesterol but Low Density Lipoproteins (LDL) are not. Low Density Lipoproteins tend to spill the cholesterol they are carrying thus depositing it in the body where it can lead to the development of plaque. Thus foods that reduce LDL and increase HDL are helpful in managing the cholesterol-induced risk of heart disease.

There is evidence that the soluble fiber found in oats, beans, fruits and vegetables, can lower cholesterol. So follow **Our recommendation** that is given in the section on Fiber:

Consume 20 - 35 grams fiber daily

*Cholesterol is simply too long a word to make a rhyming phrase that works but remember:

Cholesterol is to your arteries what hair is to your drain.

Although there has been some speculation that fish oils, in particular the omega-3 fatty acids, may have cholesterol lowering effects, this has probably been overstated. Fish is an excellent source of protein and tends to be very low in saturated fat, so it is a good food source. There is, however, no conclusive research to warrant the ingestion of omega -3 fatty acid capsules or supplements and there is some concern about their potential for misuse. In fact, the American Heart Association has recommended that fish oil capsules should not be used without medical supervision.

Make fish, not fish oil capsules, a part of your diet

Put on your dish
Not capsules but fish

Protein
Protein is the essential building block of life. It is responsible for many crucial functions in the body, like hormone production and synthesis, and cell development and function. Proteins consist of compounds called amino acids. There are 22 different amino acids and we produce 13 of

these naturally. The other nine, however, need to be come from our diet. Before you get overwhelmed by the responsibility of having to find nine essential amino acids and eat them on a daily basis, the fact is that if you eat even a moderately diverse diet you will easily fulfill your protein requirement. The biggest concern with protein is that either through fad diet or misconception, you will feel the need to eat more foods rich in protein than are necessary. Because foods that are rich in protein also tend to be high in animal fat as well, there is a danger that the drive for protein will lead you to a high fat diet.

An adult, who is not pregnant or lactating, needs approximately 0.35 grams of protein per pound body weight. Someone who is 100 pounds, therefore, needs 35 grams of protein daily. This calculates on average to about 10 - 15% calories coming from protein.

If you eat a sensible, balanced diet you will easily get enough protein. Protein is in meats, legumes, grains dairy products and a trace can be found in fruits and vegetables.

Don't use protein needs as an excuse to indulge in high-fat foods.

> **You can be lean and mean**
> **With modest protein**

Complex Carbohydrates

Complex carbohydrates are the best source of energy. While these starches contain glucose, this is different in important respects from refined sugar, and other simple sugars. Table sugar alone has no nutritional value while complex carbohydrate sugar carries with it many vitamins, minerals and other essential nutrients.

Complex carbohydrate sugar is released from the gut far more slowly than simple sugar and this maintains a more even blood-glucose level and energy flow. Fruits, vegetables, grains, cereals, breads are all good sources of complex carbohydrate.

Consume about 60 - 65% of your calories from complex carbohydrates.

Sugar, Caffeine, Sodium, Alcohol Moderation

Sugar

Sugar comes in a variety of forms. It is found in fruits in the form of fructose, for example, and this differs chemically from refined sugar or sucrose. Not only does sugar rot your teeth it influences triglycerides and mood. Other good reasons for moderating your sugar consumption include:

- Sugar calories can add up. A teaspoon of sugar in tea or coffee is 16 calories. In a typical soft drink it is 160 calories. These calories matter from a weight loss point of view.

- Many sweet foods are also very high in fat. Donuts, for example, are thought of as sugary but a typical donut is about 50% fat.

- Sugar alone has no nutritional value outside of pure energy.

- Some people seem to be primed by sugar. Once they get a taste of it they want more. It is possible that eating sweet foods leads to eating more food.

Sugar binges may leave you without energy. Although sugar will give you a quick fix in the very short term, after that energy tends to be depleted and you are left feeling lethargic.

Wherever possible use substitutes to reduce your sugar intake

Your figure will be neat
If you're food is less sweet

Caffeine

Caffeine is a drug that is found in coffee, tea, chocolate and some soft drinks. It increases nervous system arousal and increases blood flow through your kidneys. Like sugar, caffeine can stimulate you initially, but it too leads to an ultimate depletion of energy, which can leave you feeling lethargic and seeking more caffeine for increased energy.

A typical cup of coffee contains about 100 mg of caffeine. About 16% of people drinking four or more cups of coffee a day show signs of dependence. If you consume this amount, the chances are that you will become dependent on caffeine. This means that if you stop your caffeine consumption you will experience withdrawal symptoms that consist mainly of headache and extreme fatigue.

It has not been conclusively demonstrated that caffeine use is associated with serious illness. The main goal of moderating its use is to preserve energy and reduce over-arousal of your nervous system.

Consume no more than 200 mgs caffeine daily

> **It's best to wean**
> **Off too much caffeine**

Sodium

Sodium is a necessary mineral. Along with potassium and chloride, sodium acts to regulate the balance of fluids in our bodies.

We need about 500 mg sodium per day and we have to consume that amount because our body does not manufacture sodium. We can easily get that amount from natural food sources, particularly vegetables and fruits. Many people, however, consume way in excess of this amount, largely by using salt and other flavorings and buying convenience foods that are high in sodium.

Excess sodium consumption can lead to increased blood pressure and kidney problems. Even if you do not have these problems or even a family history of them, it is still advisable to be moderate in your sodium consumption and watch that salt intake. Evidence indicates that everyone responds to lower sodium intake with some reduction in their blood pressure.

Consume no more than 3000 mgs sodium daily

> **Say no, no, nodium**
> **To too much sodium**

Alcohol

Although there is some evidence that moderate alcohol consumption can be beneficial to health, these benefits can also be gained by other means, e.g. exercise, low-fat diet. Alcohol is still a potent and potentially dangerous drug. Alcohol can change your perception, the control of your behavior and it seriously impacts judgment. In addition, there are five other concerns about alcohol when considered from a wellness and weight loss point of view.

- Alcohol contains calories. Typically there about 75 calories in a glass of wine and about 150 in a 12oz beer.

- Alcohol calories are "empty" in that they have no nutritional value, except as pure energy.

- Willpower dissolves in alcohol. Once you have had a couple of drinks your perception and judgment become less reliable.

- Alcohol stimulates appetite. In conjunction with the erosion of willpower this could lead to indiscriminate and excessive eating.

- There is evidence that if you consume about 5 oz alcohol, fat storage is encouraged. This means more of your food will be stored as fat.

Have no more than 2 six ounce glasses of wine (or equivalent) on any one day

Don't drink every day

Don't drink and drive

Don't be too proud of being able to "hold your liquor." If a lot of alcohol does not seem to effect you, you are very tolerant and probably physically as well as psychologically dependent.

Women tend to tolerate alcohol less well than men and are more susceptible to alcohol-related illnesses and injury.

> **Too much liquor**
> **Will make you sicker**

Water

60% of your body weight is water, so if you weigh 180 pounds, you are carrying over 100 pounds is water! Water is more important for survival than food.

Digestion, breathing, sweating and urination deplete the body of water. If the lost water is not replaced, dehydrated occurs. Thirst is the first sign of dehydration and this begins when approximately 2% of your body water has been depleted. It is important that you do not get dehydrated so drink plenty of water before you reach this stage.

Don't wait until you get thirsty to drink. Get into the habit of drinking eight 8 ounce glasses of water daily (64 ounces total) to meet essential body requirements. Caffeinated drinks are not as good as water itself because caffeine acts as a diuretic and stimulates water loss. If you do drink a lot of caffeinated drinks remember to drink additional water to replace this extra water loss.

Drinking water can also temporarily fill you up, thus decreasing hunger and helping manage temptation.

Fiber

Fiber is not essential for human nutrition although it does seem to play a role in preventing and moderating some bowel disease and reducing cholesterol.

Fiber comes in two forms. Water-insoluble fiber, such as cellulose, hemi-cellulose and lignin, is found in whole-wheat products and fruit and vegetable skins. Water-soluble fiber, like pectin and gum, are found in fruits, vegetables, beans and oats. Fiber exerts its beneficial effect on the bowel by adding water and bulk to the stool, thus making it softer, leading to a less traumatic and faster passage through the intestine.

159

There is also evidence that soluble fiber may play role in lowering blood cholesterol levels and regulating the body's use of sugar.

Consume 20 - 35 grams fiber daily
NB: You should increase fluids as you increase your fiber intake.

Sources of Fiber		
Serving	*Food*	*Fiber (grams)*
1	Bran Muffin	4.0
1	Whole wheat bagel	2.7
2 slices	Whole-wheat bread	3.2
1 cup	Brown rice	4.5
1 oz	Wheat bran	11.3
1 oz	All Bran	8.5
1 oz	Corn Bran	5.3
1 medium	Apple	3.2
1 medium	Banana	3.0
½ cup	Blackberries	4.5
2	Dried Figs	7.4
1 medium	Orange	2.8
1 medium	Pear	4.0
5 tbsp	Raisins	3.0
½ cup	Raspberries	9.2
1 cup	Broccoli, cooked	6.5
½ cup	Green peas, cooked	2.4
½ cup	Kidney Beans, cooked	9.7
1 cup	Lentil beans, cooked	9.0
½ cup	Spinach, cooked	6.5
1 oz.	Almonds	5.0
1 oz.	Peanuts	2.5

> **Use your brains**
> **Eat plenty of grains**

Vitamins

There are 13 vitamins. Nine of these, the B vitamins and Vitamin C, are water-soluble. Vitamins A, D, E, and K are fat soluble. All of them are essential for healthy functioning. Unfortunately, because of their importance there have been too many ill-considered, unsubstantiated claims for increased intake and mega-dosing of many of these essential elements. The balance between these elements is so finely tuned that it is ill-advised to megadose on them unless specifically recommended to do so by your physician.

(The table below lists the primary function of each vitamin and some of the main sources for each. The Recommended Dietary Allowances are copyright 1989 of the National Academy of Sciences, National Academy Press, Washington D.C. The RDA's listed here are the basic ones for adults and do not refer to pregnant or lactating females, children, adolescents, or other unusual conditions.)

Vitamin B-1 (Thiamin)
Primary role: Convert carbohydrates to energy.
Sources: *Whole grains, Wheat germ, fish, peas, dried beans, soybeans, peanuts, pasta, cereal, pork*
RDA:

Adult Males	1.5 mg
Males over 50	1.2 mg
Adult Females	1.1 mg
Females over 50	1.0 mg

Vitamin B-2 (Riboflavin)
Primary role: Conversion of food to energy
Sources: *Milk, green leafy vegetables, bread, cereal, dairy products, lean meats, eggs, nuts,*
RDA:

Adult Males	1.7 mg
Males over 50	1.4 mg
Adult Females	1.3 mg
Females over 50	1.2 mg

Vitamin B-3 (Niacin)

Primary role: Energy conversion. Maintenance of skin, nerves and digestive system Doses of 3-5gms. can lower your cholesterol. Seek your physician's advice on this technique.

Sources: *Nuts, legumes, dairy products, lean meat, poultry, fish,eggs*

RDA:

Adult Males	19 mg
Males over 50	15 mg
Adult Females	15 mg
Females over 50	13 mg

Vitamin B-6 (Pyroxidine)

Primary role: Protein synthesis and immune system antibody production

Sources: *Beans, bananas, breads, eggs, fish, legumes, meats, nuts*

RDA:

Adult Males	2.0 mg
Adult Females	1.6 mg

Vitamin B-12

Primary role: Metabolism and red blood cell formation

Sources: *Eggs, milk, meat, poultry, shellfish*

RDA:

Adult Males	2.0 mcgs
Adult Females	2.0 mcgs

Vitamin B-5 (Pantothenic acid)

Primary role: Food metabolism and hormone synthesis

Sources: *Broccoli, cabbage, eggs, fish, legumes, lean beef, milk, whole-grain cereals, yeast*

RDA:

All adults	4 - 7 mg

Biotin

Primary role: Food metabolism

Sources: *Broccoli, cabbage, eggs, fish, legumes, lean beef, milk, whole-grain cereals, yeast*

RDA:

All adults	30 - 100 mcgs

Folacin

Primary role: DNA synthesis, red blood cell production
Sources: *Beans, citrus fruit, dark green leafy vegetables, pork, poultry, shellfish, wheat bran, whole grain products*
RDA:

Adult Males	**200 mcgs**
Adult females	**180 mcgs**

Vitamin C

Primary role: Maintaining healthy teeth and gums, iron absorption, keeping connective tissue healthy. There is some evidence to show that increased intake of vitamin C in the early stages of a cold reduces the duration and intensity of symptoms. Some physicians recommend doses anywhere between 500 and 4000 mgs a day. Clearly, there are individual differences and we need to know more. You should still try to get as much of your vitamin C from fruits and vegetables rather than in tablet form. The recommended dietary allowance remains at 60 mg.
Sources: *Broccoli, citrus fruits, cantaloupe, greens, potatoes, strawberries*
RDA:

All adults	**60 mg**

Vitamin A

Primary role: Promotes good vision, healthy teeth, skin, mucous membranes, skeletal and soft tissue.
Sources: *Cream, cheese, cod, kidney, liver, milk (including skim milk)*
RDA:

Adult males	**1000 mcg**
Adult females	**800 mcg**

Note: Beta Carotene, a precursor of Vitamin A, is a safer way of getting Vitamin A. Beta carotene is not toxic, whereas there is evidence that moderate to high doses of Vitamin A is.

Beta Carotene

Primary role: Protects tissue against oxidation
Sources: *Yellow orange vegetables like, carrots, pumpkins, sweet potatoes, cantaloupe, apricots*

Vitamin D:

Primary role: Absorption of calcium, maintain appropriate levels of calcium and phosphorous

Sources: *Sunlight. Various foods are fortified with vitamin D, like butter, cheese, cream, margarine, all milk, oysters, fortified cereals*

RDA:

Males to 25 years	**10 mcg**
Males over 26	**5 mcg**
Females to 25 years	**10 mcg**
Females over 26	**5 mcg**

Vitamin E:

Primary role: Protects tissues against oxidation, red blood cell formation

Sources: *Asparagus, corn, nuts, seeds, olives, vegetable oils (except palm and coconut oil), spinach, wheat germ*

RDA:

Adult males	**10 mg**
Adult females	**8 mg**

Vitamin K:

Primary role: Coagulation of blood

Sources: *Cabbage, cauliflower, cereals, spinach, soybean oil.*

RDA:

Adult males to 25 years	**65 mcg**
Adult males over 26	**80 mcg**
Adult females to 25 years	**55 mcg**
Adult females over 26 years	**65 mcg**

Antioxidants

There is some evidence that Vitamin C, Vitamin E and Beta Carotene, the so-called anti-oxidants, have a beneficial effect on health by neutralizing "free radicals."

Free radicals are charged subatomic particles that are the natural bi-product of oxidation. Well controlled studies have shown that daily use of ant-oxidants produced:

40% reduction in cancer

30% reduction in heart attacks

The study was done using the following daily doses

Vitamin C 1000 mg

Vitamin E 400 units

Beta Carotene   25,000 units

Other studies have demonstrated reduction in cataracts, reduced injury from excessive exercise, and reduction of exercise-related stiffness and soreness.

Dr. England, the family physician adviser to the *7 Steps To Wellness* program says that Vitamin C can be helpful in treating and preventing routine recurrent urinary tract infections. Most urinary pathogens grow better in an alkaline environment and vitamin C at 1000 mg/day will usually drop the urinary pH several points and help suppress bacterial growth.

Dr. England also suggests that during the duration of a common cold you should take 3000 - 4000 mgs of Vitamin C in divided doses of 1000 mg taken three or four times a day. For children over two, Dr England recommends a daily dose100 mg of Vitamin C per year of age with a maximum of 2000 mgs for pre-adolescents. For children, Vitamin C is available in 100mg, 250 mg and 500 mg tablets, and the dose should be divided every six hours during the duration of the common cold. Divided doses are advised because vitamin C has a half-life of only four to six hours. There are some contraindications to anti-oxidants supplementation.

People with a history of kidney stones should avoid vitamin C supplementation.

People with abnormal bleeding tendency should avoid Vitamin E supplementation as it may prolong bleeding.

With these exceptions in mind, Dr England routinely recommends daily anti-oxidant supplementation for all non-pregnant adults.

Recent studies suggest that smokers may have increased health risks if they take Beta carotene in the doses recommended above. So the second most important recommendation to a smoker is to avoid taking Beta carotene. Of course, the most important recommendation to a smoker is - STOP SMOKING NOW!

**A multivitamin a day
Keeps your HMO at bay**

<u>**Managing Portion Size**</u>
Portion size is an important part of eating a healthy diet. If you are minimizing the amount of fat in your diet, you are going to be eating healthily. If you are just trying to eat healthily and not lose weight, you can probably eat a lot of non-fat foods (watch the sugar content, 'though). Because non-fat foods have only 4 calories per gram (compared to the 9 calories in a fat gram), they are not going to be a big factor in *weight maintenance*. **If you are trying to lose weight however, the overall number of calories consumed is a factor and you will need to watch overall calorie intake as well as fat grams. Simple ways of managing portion size are:**

> Use small plates
> Start with small portions (you can always get more)
> Split entrees
> Make a meal out of appetizers
> Order half-portions or even seniors or children's servings

166

Specify specific portion sizes
Drink fluids with meal (watch the alcohol!)

Nutrition Quiz
(Circle the appropriate answer)
The 7% solution means that I will get no more than what percentage of my calories from saturated fat?

5%   7%   9%   11%   13%

How many calories are there in a gram of fat?

4   40   9   90   900

You should not exceed what percentage of calories in you total diet from unsaturated fats?

4%   10%   15%   20%   25%

The maximum recommended daily intake of caffeine is

100mgs 200mgs 500mgs 100 gms

The recommended daily intake of fiber is about

10gms 25 gms 50 gms 100 gms

The percentage of your diet that should be in the form of complex carbohydrates is

20%   40%   60%   80%   99%

Answers below[17]

---

[17] Answers: 7%, 9, 15%, 200mgs., 25 grams, 60%

Exercise

A Crucial Component of a Wellness Program

Exercise has so many benefits that it is a key component to any a weight loss and wellness effort. If you were to adopt one new behavior that would improve your health and well-being it would be developing an exercise program (unless you are a smoker, where quitting is your number one priority).

The most important behavior in a successful weight loss program is walking! If you do this one activity you are more than half way to achieving your weight management goals.

There is no other single behavior that can give you all of the advantages listed below. How much would you pay for a drug that gave you all of these benefits?

Increased longevity
Increase quality of life
Increased stamina and endurance
Increased feeling of well-being
Increased energy
Increase in metabolism
Reduced risk of heart disease
Reduced risk of cancer
Burns calories
Lowers harmful cholesterol
Increases good cholesterol
Improved management of stress
Increased immune system function
Tones muscle
Preserves muscle mass
Preserves bone
Improves mood

A regular, sensible exercise program can provide you with all of the above. This is not hype. The benefits listed above have been demonstrated scientifically so many times that it is not funny.

I know the word "exercise" might fill you full of apprehension and even loathing, but the fact is that the benefits listed above are easier to come by than you imagine. You might even to get to enjoy it!

What do I mean exactly when I say "exercise"? There are various forms of exercise that are beneficial but at its simplest exercise means moving your muscles. Proper exercise will improve flexibility, cardiovascular fitness and strength.

There are three main principles in developing fitness.

1. **Specificity.** To achieve certain benefits (e.g. improved muscle mass) specific exercises are needed (e.g. resistance exercises). No one exercise can meet all your exercise needs.

2. **Overload.** The body, like the mind, develops when it has to adapt to manageable overload. When this overload is slowly and progressively increased, fitness improves. The three dimensions of overload are

> Frequency - The number of times the exercise is performed

> Intensity - Adaptation and improved fitness occur when the exercise gradually increases in intensity

> Duration - The amount of time spent doing the exercise is another overload variable.

3. **Reversibility.** Sensible, regular exercise will improve fitness. Fitness levels will decrease, however, if those exercise routines are not maintained.

There are three different types of exercise:

> **Aerobic type** activity for cardiovascular conditioning, calorie burning and energy.
> **Stretching exercises** for flexibility

Resistance exercises for strength development and endurance

Aerobic type activity
Aerobic activity involves constant movement that increases heart rate. Aerobic technically means getting your heart rate to a particular range.

The formula for working out the lower limit of the aerobic range is:

220 - age x 0.6

So, if you are forty years old, the lower limit is
220 - 40 = 180

180 x 0.6 = 108

The lower limit of a forty-year old's aerobic range is therefore a heart rate of 108 beats per minute.

The upper limit on your range is

220 - age x 0.75

So for a forty year-old the upper limit on their aerobic range is:
220 - 40 = 180

180 x 0.75 = 135

The upper limit on your aerobic range is 135 beats per minute.

So, for a forty year-old, the range on a good aerobic workout is 108 to 135 beats per minute.

This does not mean, however, that you cannot have periods that exceed 135 beats per minute (or whatever your upper aerobic limit is). If you are particularly fit and want to get into top-notch physical condition, short training periods (about 10% of total exercise time) in excess of 135 may be beneficial. For this level of fitness seek the help of a trained professional.

> ### *Seeking Medical Advice Before Exercising*
> *Although most people can quite safely increase their activity levels without undue medical concern, the following groups should consult a physician before embarking on an exercise program:*
>
> *If you have a family history or suffered from symptoms of cardiovascular disease, hypertension, diabetes, lung or kidney disease, atherosclerosis*
>
> *If you are very unfit and have been very sedentary*
>
> *If you are a female over 50*
>
> *If you are a male over 40*
>
> *If you are a heavy smoker*
>
> *If you are already under medical supervision*
>
> *If you are overweight*

Do not worry excessively about aerobic numbers. For one thing, a variety of factors interfere with this calculation, like medication.

More importantly, though, **it is not necessary to even be aerobically active to receive substantial benefits from exercise.** It is true that aerobic activity will give your heart a good work-out but you can get a good work-out without being aerobic. More importantly, however, you will probably get close to your aerobic range if you get into any activity that requires constant movement and you do it at a brisk pace.

The effort required to get aerobic is determined by your level of fitness. If you are very unfit, even the lightest exercise is likely to increase your heart rate into the aerobic range, whereas if you are already fit you are going to work much harder to get aerobic. That is why you should exercise with people of similar fitness levels to you.

There are several types of aerobic activity.

Walking
Swimming
Jogging
Cycling
Water aerobics
Cross country skiing
Rope skipping

Aerobics classes vary in difficulty and quality. Get an instructor who is qualified, is concerned about making sure the participants are exercising appropriately and can accommodate different fitness levels in class members.

Step aerobics use a step to increase the difficulty of the work-out.

Low-Impact aerobics use exercises that minimize the stress on joints.

Duration
Aerobic exercise should last at least twenty minutes. There is some evidence to suggest this exercise can be divided into smaller segments. For example, instead of walking for thirty minutes, walk three times for ten minutes. This is more of a practical matter. If you can exercise for the allotted time all in one go, I would encourage you to do that. It is more likely that you will get the exercise done in this way. It is comforting to know, however, that even if you do not have a block of time, breaking it down into smaller segments is still effective.

Frequency
You should plan to do aerobic exercise between three and five times a week.

Training effect
Aerobic capacity can be improved by increasing the amount of time spent exercising or the pace. With continued aerobic workouts, heart rate will not get as high while working out at the initial level and harder work (e.g. walk faster and/or longer) will be more easily tolerated. Resting heart rate will also be reduced.

172

Assessment: Walk one mile as fast as you can without straining. Record your time. That will be your base time. You can do this test once every couple of weeks, initially, to monitor your improvement.

Goals: Use your performance on the assessment test to set goals for aerobic activity. For example, if you walked the mile in thirty minutes, retest yourself in a month with the goal of reducing your one mile time to twenty-five minutes.

Choice: Although walking is likely to be your aerobic activity of choice, don't forget the other activities that you could do for variety. Variety is important - it reminds you of other activities and prevents boredom.

The aerobic-type activity that most people use, however, is walking. This is natural, requires no special equipment, can be done anywhere and is something you don't have to think about.

Make walking the foundation of your exercise program.

Other activities include bicycling, both stationary and regular, and swimming -- although note that swimming tends not to be the best activity from a calorie burning, weight loss point of view. Other activities like tennis, golf and other competitive sports, are typically not aerobic because they do not involve constant movement. There is too much stopping and starting for these sports to confer aerobic type advantages but they are excellent additions to a regular exercise program.

Here are the current recommendations as far as aerobic-type activity is concerned:

- Always warm-up first and cool-down immediately after your routine (see box)

- If you are just starting an exercise program, begin with walking 15 - 20 minutes at a time and progressively work up to thirty minutes over a period of 4 - 6 weeks.

- Do your exercise for no less than thirty minutes a day. You can break this up, into say 10 minutes three times a day, but in my experience most people prefer to do it all at once.

- Exercise for a minimum of three times a week. Five times a week is ideal.

- Vary your routine and activity to prevent boredom.

- Don't waste your money on fitness gimmicks, or exercise equipment unless you know for a *cast-iron, absolute fact*, you will use them. Instead, spend at least $50 on a proper pair of walking or other exercise shoes.

Warming up:
It is important to slowly warm your body up before exercising. A warm-up routine of slow stretches (no bouncing, please), helps improve bloodflow. Do not overstretch. For walking start off slowly and gradually increase the pace.

Cooling down:
It is important to slow your system down gradually. Never stop exercising abruptly, always ease into it by reducing your pace slowly.

Now, as a sign of your commitment to yourself, sign the following form.

I commit to walk for at least fifteen minutes a day, at least three times a week for the next four weeks.

Signed..

Date............................

The Perceived Exertion Scale
This scale measures how hard you are working out.. The seven points on the scale are:
Very easy
Easy
Somewhat easy

Moderate
Somewhat Difficult
Difficult
Very Difficult

Keep yourself in the "moderate" range and never get above "somewhat difficult."

If you are exercising so hard that you cannot hold a conversation you are exercising too intensely.

Stretching
The purpose of flexibility exercises is to tone muscle and to keep supple. There are various types of stretching exercises, including yoga. These exercises develop better muscular and body control.

Duration
Initially, hold a stretch for ten seconds. With practice, you will be able to hold a stretch comfortably for up to sixty seconds. Never stretch beyond the point of discomfort.

Frequency
A flexibility workout should be done three times a week.

Training effect
Improved muscle tone and body control will result from regular flexibility exercises.

Assessment. Flexibility is specific to each joint so there are no general flexibility tests. A common test is the sit-and -reach which rates flexibility of the lower back. The standing-toe-touch rates flexibility of hamstrings.

Goal: To increase overall flexibility

Choice: Static stretching in which a muscle is stretched gradually and held it for between 10 to 60 seconds is best. This slow movement helps to safely stretch farther than usual.

Ballistic stretching, in which muscles are stretched suddenly in a bouncing motion **should be avoided** because it can cause injury.

For each static stretch, slowly stretch to the point of slight tension and hold the position for ten to sixty seconds. As the tension declines, stretch a little bit farther. Rest 30-60 seconds between each stretch and repeat three to five time for each.

The best stretching routine is one that is done slowly and where you hold the stretch to the point at which you feel resistance and not beyond.

Flexibility exercises are designed to stretch muscles. This will develop flexibility and a degree of muscle strength. Simple stretching exercises can prevent the build-up of muscle tension and stiffness.

Stretching exercises have been shown to be beneficial to groups of all ages. Increased flexibility will not only make you feel better but reduces the chance of muscle injury. Stretching exercises are helpful in preparing for more vigorous activity and should always be used as part of a warm-up routine.

As a minimum, you should do stretching exercises at least three times a week. As part of a basic stretching routine, I suggest five simple exercises that require no special equipment and about ten minutes of your time.

The Rules of the Static Stretching Routine

- Always warm-up. Warm-up should consist of gentle movement lasting about five minutes. Walk on the spot slowly or gently move arms and legs.

- Discontinue the stretch if you feel pain.

- Do not bounce.

- Hold the stretch only until you feel resistance. **Never hold the stretch beyond the point of discomfort.**

- Maintain regular breathing through the stretch. Do not hold your breath while stretching.

- Keep your body aligned. Do not arch your back.

- Do not overtax joints.

The five basic stretches are:

Calf Stretch:
Stand facing a wall from about two or three feet. Lean forward against the wall ensuring that your rear heel stays on the floor. Hold the stretch until you feel the beginnings of resistance or discomfort. Repeat twice for each leg.

Thigh stretch:
Holding hand against the wall, hold left (right) ankle in left (right) hand and pull your feet towards your waist. Hold the stretch until you feel the beginnings of resistance or discomfort. Twice for each leg. Keep your back straight.

Outer thigh stretch:
Holding hand against wall, place left foot behind and outside of right foot. Bend left ankle and lean towards the wall. Hold the stretch until you feel the beginnings of resistance or discomfort. Repeat twice for each leg.

Hamstring stretch:
Lie on floor with knees bent. With both hands, pull your right leg towards your chest. Straighten leg and hold the stretch until you feel the beginnings of resistance or discomfort. Slowly lower leg. Repeat twice for each leg.

Lower back stretch:
Lie on floor with hands behind knees. Gradually pull both knees forward towards chest, keeping back pressed against the floor. Hold the stretch until you feel the beginnings of resistance or discomfort. Relax and repeat twice more.

Do your stretch routine at least once, three times a week.

Stretch during the day to ward off muscle tension and stiffness.

As you get into the habit of doing your stretching routine, you may want increase the amount of time that you hold the stretch. You can increase the time up to thirty seconds, but remember only to hold the stretch until you feel the beginnings of resistance and discomfort. As you increase your flexibility you may want to add other flexibility exercises including the following..

Hip flexor stretch
From kneeling position move left foot forward so that chin, knee and ankle are aligned. Keep right knee on the floor and the left foot straight. Using hands on floor for support lean gently forward to create hip flexor stretch. Hold the stretch until you feel the beginnings of resistance or discomfort. Repeat and then switch legs.

Lower Back stretch
Lay flat on the floor with arms outstretched. Bend left leg so knee is at 90 degrees and with right arm gently pull left knee over right leg. Keep head on floor facing outstretched arm, shoulders flat against the floor. Keep head facing outstretched arm. Hold the stretch until you feel the beginnings of resistance or discomfort.

Don't be a wretch
Give those muscles a stretch

Strength Training
Resistance exercises for strength development
Resistance exercises are an other essential part of your wellness program. Resistance exercises, which involve training against a resistance will stress muscle and bone. This type of activity help preserve, as well as build, lean muscle mass. Lean muscle mass is what determines your metabolic rate and it is crucial that you preserve it. If you don't, your metabolic rate will drop and you have an increased risk of weight gain.

Muscular Strength and Endurance

Assessment of muscular strength: What is the heaviest weight you can lift just one time?

Assessment of muscular endurance; Count the maximum number of contraction repetitions (as in push-up or sit-up) or the maximum time a muscle contraction (e.g. bicep curl) can be held.

Goals: A complete muscular strength program works all the major muscle groups including upper back, shoulders, arms, chest, abdomen, low back, thighs, buttocks and calves.

By using weights that are as heavy as 80% of your maximum capacity you can build strength. For example, if the heaviest weight you can lift is currently ten pounds, a good starting to weight would be 8 pounds.

For muscular *endurance*, a good weight is about 50% of maximum capacity (i.c. 5 pounds if the maximum weight you can lift is 10 pounds). As strength (and maximum capacity) increase, use heavier weights.

This type of strength training routine is concerned with preserving muscle. This is not body building! Resistance exercises stress bone and help keep it healthy, an important factor for seniors, particularly senior women at risk for osteoporosis. **Resistance exercises are great for both women and men and for all ages.**

There are five simple resistance exercises at the core of my strength training routine. Three of these core exercises require some light ankle weights.

The rules of strength training.

- Always warm up with simple stretching or gentle movement.

- Work slowly

- Stop if you feel any pain.

- Cool down by repeating warm-up routine.

The five basic exercises are:

Abdominals:
Sit on the floor, knees bent, feet flat on the floor. Gently lower yourself to the floor. use your arms to push yourself back up. Repeat five to ten times.
Total time: 1 -2 minutes

Heel raises:
Stand with the balls of your feet resting on a book. Gradually rise on your toes then gently lower your heels as far as you can. You might need to use your hands for balance.
Total time: 1 minute

Quadriceps:
With light ankle weights attached sit up on a desk, table or stool. Gradually straighten one knee. Keeping your back straight and your foot flexed. Hold for five seconds. Gradually lower, repeat then switch.
Total time: 1 minute

Hamstrings:
With ankle weight attached, hold on to chair for support. Gradually lift your heel towards your buttocks. Lower gradually. Repeat then switch to other leg.
Total time: 1 minute

Toe raises:
With ankle weight attached sit on stool. Gradually raise the ball of your foot and then lower. Repeat then switch to other foot.
Total time: 1 minute

There are other, more advanced exercises, that do require the purchase of a set of weights.

The rules of exercising with weights.
* Start with light weights that you can lift comfortably from eight to fifteen times (This is called a set.)

- As you gain strength, you can increase the number of repetition (up to fifteen) or increase the weight.

- If you work the same muscle group for consecutive sets, you need to rest for about two minutes between each set. This does not apply if you are exercising different muscle groups.

- Work gradually and smoothly.

- Make a conscious effort to breathe out when you lift. It is tempting to hold your breath when lifting but this can lead to problems, notably a rapid increase in blood pressure.

- As with any form of exercise, stop immediately if you feel any pain. The idea is to temporarily fatigue the muscle groups you are working on, not to feel pain.

- Do not forget to cool down with a few stretches.

Further strength training exercises

Bench fly
Lying on a raised surface hold weights straight up over your chest, your elbows slightly bent. Gradually lower the weights until they are level with your chest. Then life them slowly back up to the starting position over your chest. Repeat from eight to fifteen times.

Lateral raise
Stand in the "neutral" position (Knees slightly bent, legs about shoulder width apart, weight evenly distributed, toes to the front). Start with weights at thigh level and gradually lift them out to the sides until they are at shoulder height. Keep elbows bent. Lower gradually and repeat eight to fifteen times.

Upright row
From the "neutral" position hold weights together at thigh level, palms inward. Gradually lift the weights in front of you until they reach just above shoulder height. Lower gradually and repeat eight to fifteen times.

Bicep curls

From the "neutral" position, stand with weight at your side, palms towards you. Gradually lift weights to your shoulders then lower slowly. Repeat eight to fifteen times.

Tricep lift

From the "neutral" position, stand with weight in one hand, elbow bent, weight level with your ear. Gradually extend arm straight up so that weight is above your head. gradually lower. Repeat then switch arms.

Do a strength training work-out three times a week.

> **A little hustle**
> **Preserves your muscle**

Making Exercise Happen

Here are ten pointers that I have found to be the most useful in helping people begin and maintain a good exercise program.

1. Choose an activity that is natural to you.

Ski machines are great for skiers, and rowing machines are great for rowers and bicycles are great for bikers but if you don't do these things already it is unlikely that they will form the basis of an enduring exercise regime. It is this reason that makes **walking** a popular and successful choice for many people.

> **Most people know how to walk, but it's tough to row and chew gum at the same time**

2. Make a commitment to exercise.

At least commit to exercise four times a week for the next four weeks.

> **Each time you make the effort to exercise, you're not just moving you are reaffirming your commitment to yourself**

3. Make an appointment with yourself to exercise.

Write it down in your diary - it is as important as any other appointment you have -- so don't pre-empt it. You cannot afford to wing it -- to mentally make a loose commitment to exercise on a particular day. You need to be committed.

Exercise is an appointment with yourself that you have to keep

---

Exercise Appointment Time:Part A
I am going to walk on the following days (circle at least three)
Monday   Tuesday   Wednesday   Thursday   Friday
    Saturday   Sunday

I am going to take my walk at the following times (circle the closest appropriate time)

In the mornings at: 6 7 8 9 10 11 12noon
In the afternoons/evenings at: 1 2 3 4 5 6 7 8

While I am walking I am going to
    Listen to music
    Listen to other audiotapes
    Daydream
    Think creatively

Signed.. Date........................

---

4. Make a commitment to do something.

Even if that means just going out of the door for thirty seconds and coming back again. Always do something.

A little bit of something is better than a large part of nothing

---

5. Create a particular time and routine for your exercise.
Establishing a routine is important.

The journey of a thousand miles begins with putting on your sneakers

6. Keep your exercise clothes handy.
If you exercise first thing in the morning have them right there, roll into them and head out the door.

The easier a behavior is, the more likely you are to do it

7. Eliminate interruptions.

If you are working out at home, put the answer machine on, do not answer the door, do not arrange for people to be coming by the house, for whatever reason, during your scheduled exercise time.

Do not make it easy for you to be deflected from your exercise schedule

---

8. Make exercise enjoyable.

Keep yourself amused while excrcising. Physical activity like walking does not require any attention, which frees your mind up to think of other things. Listen to your favorite music, or books on tape, or other audiotapes, or watch television or videotapes. You can also use your exercise time to daydream and think creatively.

Do not use your mind to time your exercise, use your time to exercise your mind.

---

9. Roam.

Outside of scheduled exercise time, take the opportunity for physical exercise. Take the stairs rather than the elevator, park a little farther away and walk, take more stretch breaks during the day. Remember, every calorie counts!

The climb to success in wellness begins with taking the stairs rather than the elevator

---

Special tip: PHONE WALKING. Got a portable phone? If you have, just walk (up and down or around and around) while you are on the phone. You will burn hundreds of calories more that way.

10. Notice how good you feel

Focus on how good you feel after you have exercised. See, how long those effects last. Compare your feelings on days when you do and don't exercise.

> No matter how bad you feel before hand, exercise will always make you feel better

WARNING! You do not have to sweat and pant to get benefit from exercise. In fact, it you feel discomforted in any way, you should stop. A good rule of thumb is: If you are exerting yourself so hard you cannot hold a conversation, you are working too hard.

Stop exercising immediately if:

You feel pain

You have chest pain or pressure

You have pain in your neck, jaw or arm

You feel dizzy or light-headed

You feel nauseated

You have blurred vision

You have severe breathlessness

You feel faint

If you experience these symptoms report to a physician

If you do get injured or suffer pain in joints, seek the advice of a sports physician.

Weight Management and Wellness For All
10 Great Ways to Shape Up Your Spouse and Your Family

1: Set Modest, Simple Health goals.
If your spouse is completely sedentary don't expect him/her to begin a full blown exercise program just because you ask. But suggest going for a five minute walk together after meals, a couple of times a week. A walk is a great time to talk, but don't make it too heavy. People will only repeat behaviors they find enjoyable. Once you have established the habit of going for short walk, you can build from there.

Your kids are not going to give up french fries, ice-cream and chocolate just because you ask. You can, however, slowly introduce healthier foods, like pasta and fruit, or simply slowly increase the amount of healthy food they already like. You can give them low-fat or fat-free alternatives for treats **without even mentioning their fat content or their nutritional value.** Use some of Colleen's great recipes that come with this program and your family won't even know they are eating healthier! Remember the purpose here is to get your family into healthier habits not give them a Ph.D. in nutrition and exercise physiology.

Be content with any progress no matter how slow the process may seem to you.

2: Reinforce Healthy Behavior
Your sedentary spouse agrees to go for a ten minute walk. After five minutes he/she says, "I've got to get back now because there's that great program on TV." While your initial reaction will probably be one of frustration or even anger, focus on the fact that he walked five minutes more than he normally would, not that he cut it short. If you create a conflict out of it, you may never get him walking again.

You prepare a healthy meal for your child who normally only eats a high-fat diet with no fruits or vegetables. They complain about half the meal but eat the rest including some of the good stuff. Don't get into a battle about what they didn't eat - be pleased with a little progress. Conflict will only polarize. React positively.

Always acknowledge effort and progress even if it's not as much as what you wanted.

3: Focus on Motivation

As men get into their forties and beyond, their main motivation for lifestyle change comes from a desire to "get back into shape" and to avoid ill health. Capitalize on this wherever possible. Scan the obituaries for news about men dying young (even better if they are the same age as your spouse). Try to be subtle about this. Do not tape the obit to your husband's cereal bowl but just leave the paper lying around with a noticeable asterisk next to the appropriate column. If challenged about it, simply tell your husband that you are not yet ready to see his obituary in the paper.

Children are motivated by all sorts of things; a desire to make the team, join the group or impress an individual. Your children's idols, be they sports heroes, rock stars or movie personalities are typically fit and in shape. They have to be to meet their demands of being at the top of their profession. You might not like the hair color or cut of your son's favorite basketball hero but that basketball player is definitely in shape and you can use this fact to help motivate your child.

Understand what motivates your family and use it to get them on track

4: Go Public

The anticipation of being in a public place can be a great motivator. The desire to look good and perform well (or at the very least not embarrass oneself) at a future public event can provide a good short term goal.

You might, for example, get your partner to agree to join you in the charity walk that the hospital is staging. Your partner will soon realize, without you having to tell him/her, that he/she will not want to embarrass himself by huffing and puffing by the side of the road as he is overtaken by walkers who are twice his/her age. The idea of a little training has thus been planted and you're off and running -- well, walking.

Social pressure is a particularly useful motivation tool for children. If there is a big event in their future you can use this as motivation but

188

sensitive about appearance. But remember, a healthy lifestyle is not just about looks -- it's about feeling good and performing at your peak. You can use a desire to do well in upcoming exams just as easily as a desire to look good at the prom as a motivator.

Social pressure is a very powerful influence

5. Associate Health with Favorite Activities
Your spouse loves golf, or hunting and fishing or even shopping. Any activity can be performed better when you can move more easily and freely. Use the idea of improved performance at activities that are already valued as a motivator for at least a little exercise, or better nutrition, or more relaxation. Your kids want to be the best cheerleader, football player, guitarist. They are more likely to reach these goals if they are in shape, mentally and physically.

People repeat behaviors they find enjoyable

6. Exert Influence not Control
The trick to effectively influencing people is to make them feel as if the decision for action is theirs. Even if it isn't their idea, they need to think that it is. If they don't own it, they won't do it.

Your spouse is concerned about being out of shape but has not yet been moved to action. You know that direct discussion makes them sensitive and defensive. So don't address it with them directly. Talk about other people you know who are out of shape and suffering the consequences. Talk about other people who are in shape and reaping the benefits. Wonder out loud whether that public figure who just dropped dead of a heart attack at the age of 42 really could have avoided his fate with lifestyle change, and if so, why he didn't. Be subtle.

Likewise, lead your children to the idea of healthier action don't force it down their throat.

Lead a horse to water and it will drink. Order a horse to water and it will die of thirst.

7. Lead by Example

The best way of influencing people is to lead by example. If you are eating healthily and exercising sensibly and your family can see the benefits, there is a much greater chance that they will follow suit. The worst thing you can do is preach one thing, but do another, especially with children.

Each time you make healthy decisions and take healthy actions you are influencing your family.

8. Make It Easy for Your Family to be Healthy

Don't obstruct any attempt to be healthier.

Your partner is about to slump onto the sofa after dinner. You say, "I'm just going out for a short walk, do you want to come?" Even better, you might disguise the whole idea more subtly with something like, "You ought to see the house that they're building at the end of the street! I am just going to check it out."

Your normally sedentary child wants to go play soccer for the first time with the neighborhood kids. Don't tell him he can't go until he cleans up his room or has dinner or puts the dog back together again.

Only obstruct a healthy activity if absolutely necessary

9. Negotiate

Do not be shy about negotiating healthy behaviors with your family.

Your husband wants to watch the play-offs. You offer to let him watch the game in a guilt free peace providing he takes a walk with you at half-time, or before the game, and/or eats only one small bag of fat-free chips during it (the game that is, not the walk).

Your child wants to dye his hair green. Suggest that eating green foods might have the same effect and save the cost of the dye. Negotiate acceptance of green hair only after he has tried a diet that includes green foods like broccoli, spinach, lettuce, kiwi, fruit, etc.

Wheeling and dealing can bring physical healing

10. Do Activities Together.

Your family is the most important aspect of your life. Your mutual desire to be healthy and performing at your peak is a reflection of your love for each other. Togetherness and love should characterize all of your activities, including the drive for health and wellness. So make sure that you plan to be active together, whether that is sweeping the leaves, walking the neighborhood or spring cleaning the house.

A family that walks together, talks together.

Appendix A: Avoiding Known Risks

While we only know about some of the risks to our wellness it is important that we take precautionary steps against known hazards in our life.

One of those hazards is our genes which do predispose us towards a particular health profile and it is unwise (sometimes suicidal) to ignore these factors. Your family history, along with your age and any symptoms you have experienced, determine the type and frequency of medical screening.

Listed below are the current advisories for medical screening for the adult population covering the most common conditions. Remember an ounce or prevention is worth a pound of cure. Actually, the ratio is far greater for prevention: early detection is the key to survival.

The other risks are implicit in our lifestyle. There are simple behaviors that can protect you from accidents and illness and substantially improve your chances of a long and high-quality life.

I've listed some of the known risks below, with simple advice on how to avoid the perils implicit in them.

Sexually Transmitted Diseases
- Have single partner relationships
- Know the physical condition and sexual practices of your sexual partners
- Use spermicidal jellies
- Use latex condoms

Car Accidents
- Don't drink and drive
- Don't drive while taking any medications that make you drowsy
- Don't drive while fatigued
- If you're sleepy pull off the road until you have revived
- Wear seat belts

- Ensure children are in appropriate seat belts/restrainers
- Don't drive too fast
- Don't tailgate
- Slow down in poor weather
- Pay attention - don't read or make long phonecalls
- Keep your vehicle well maintained.

Accidents at home

Don't operate machinery or dangerous equipment, including guns, if:

- You are not trained in their use
- You are fatigued
- You have been drinking alcohol or illicit drugs
- You are withdrawing from alcohol or drugs
- You are not feeling well
- You are not paying attention

- Wear safety goggles and protective clothing
- Install fire alarms and smoke detectors
- Use fire guards
- Install nonskid bathmats in and by the side of tubs/ showers
- Don't leave objects lying about on stairs or floors
- Keep high traffic areas well lit

Screening and Examinations

Self-examination

Early detection is the best chance of successful treatment. It is, therefore, important that you get in the habit of looking for changes in your body. It is also very important to report any changes immediately to a physician.

Do not be embarrassed to seek medical advice when you think that a symptom is only a minor abnormality or not even an abnormality at all. If your physician makes you feel embarrassed when you do, change your physician.

Do not be dismissive of physical changes. You are not medically qualified—you don't know, it could be serious. Seeking help will do two great things for you. It will either put your mind at rest or get you help at the earliest possible time.

Any changes in your body should be a cause for further examination and analysis. Be especially watchful for any lumps, moles or skin alterations that occur. Any blood that appears in stools, urine or sputum should be reported. Changes in bowel habits also should be followed closely unless they reflect an obvious change in dietary practice.

Scheduled examinations

Recommended check-ups for adults by medical professionals
Recommended check-ups are designed to screen for normal function and detect any signs of disease.

Eye examination:
High risk category: *Symptoms, or family history of, diabetes, hypertension, glaucoma*
Frequency of test: *Annually or as physician recommends*

Not high risk category:
Frequency of test: *Every 2 years*

Dental Examination
High risk category: Smokers and tobacco chewers
Frequency of test: *Annually or as physician recommends*

Not high risk category:
Frequency of test: *At least once a year*

Cervical (Pap) smear
High risk category: *Women who have symptoms or family history of cervical cancer, or have herpes, genital warts*
Frequency of test: *Annually or as physician recomends*

Not high risk category:
Frequency of test: *Every 1-3 years under 50: Every 3-5 years over 50*

Blood Pressure check:

High risk category: *Symptoms, or family histotry of,hypertension, heart disease,kidney disease, stroke, diabetes and/or those who are obese or are taking an oral contraceptive*
Frequency of test: *Annually or as physician recomends*

Not high risk category:
Frequency of test: *Every 3 years under 50: Every year over 50*

Cholesterol test:

High risk category:*Symptoms, or family history of, coronary heart disease, hypercholesteremia*
Frequency of test: *Annually or as physician recommends*

Not high risk category:
Frequency of test: *Every 3 years*

Mammogram:

High risk category: *Symptoms, or family history of, breast cancer*
Frequency of test: *Annually or as physician recommends*

Not high risk category:
Frequency of test: *Every 1-2 years under 50: Every year after 50*

Rectal and colon examinations:

High risk category: *Symptoms, or family history, of colo-rectal cancer, chronic ulcerative colitis, or colonic polyps*
Frequency of test: *Annually or as physician recommends*

Not high risk category:
Frequency of test: *Every year after 40*

Complete physical examination

Every 1-2 years under 65; Every year after 65.

The Meal Plan

As you preview your menu you will note the days are numbered instead of in a calendar fashion. This was done for those people who have a hard time starting their week . There are a few comments to be made. If you do not like some of the suggested foods you may substitute from within the same food group. Note the diet is high in fiber and low in fat. If you have a cholesterol problem I suggest you use egg substitutes when eggs are used. You can see the amount of fat, salt, and cholesterol content for each day at the bottom of the menu.

When salads are mentioned you are required to use at least 1 cup of lettuce. You may use more if you would like, but you are limited to the amount of dressing, However, you can use vinegar freely on your salads. If the flavor is bland you may use either Spike or Vegit seasoning to season your vegetables or entrees.

I hope you enjoy the menu and good luck with your results!

Colleen Wracker R.D.

Grocery Lists

The following is a master grocery list for week one and week two. This will help with meal preparation. You will notice week one is longer because most of the recipes are made that week. So week two you can enjoy some left-overs.

To help with planning , I suggest you make the recipes according to directions and pre-portion them out and freeze immediately. This will save the flavor at its peak as long as it is eaten with in 1 month of freezing. That is, if it is stored appropriately.

Some items on the list can be frozen also even though you may have bought them fresh or in the refrigerated section. I recommend the following: tortillas, luncheon meats, bagels, muffins, rolls, hamburger buns, and meats.

Week I

Fruits
small can or jar of applesauce
1 cantaloupe
1 large can of peaches in lite syrup
2 apples of any variety
1 small can of apricots in lite syrup
2 lbs. grapes red or white, seedless
1 large can tropical fruit
1 pink grapefruit
1 small can pineapple in lite syrup

Vegetables
bunch romaine lettuce
1 bunch leaf lettuce
10 tomatoes, medium
1 small bag baby carrots
1 yellow squash
1 zucchini
1 red pepper
1 stalk celery
2 bunches parsley
8oz. white mushrooms
1 bunch green onions
1 lb. white onions
2 yellow or green or red peppers
1 purple or sweet onion
6oz. portabella or cremmini mushroons
1 lb. bag whole carrots
1 bell pepper
3 10oz. pkg. frozen spinach
1 10oz. frozen broccoli
1 lb. fresh broccoli
1 10oz. frozen green beans
1 10oz. frozen carrots
1 10oz. frozen mixed vegetable
1 6oz. frozen pea pods
14oz. stir fry vegetables
2 16oz. cans mixed vegetables

Grains

	Calorie	Fat	Serving
1 bag raisin cinnamon bagels	200	1	item
1 oat bran english muffins	150	1	item
1 box whole wheat crackers	60-80	0-3	5
1 box frozen pancakes	180	2	item
1 loaf whole wheat bread	80-110	1	item
1 bag whole wheat rolls, small size	80-110	1	item
2 low fat muffins, fresh or frozen	140-150	3	item
1 lb. brown rice, long grain	130-150	1	1/2 c
1 lb. tricolor pasta	210	1	2 oz
1/2 lb. wild rice	210	1	1/2c
1 box frozen waffles	150-175	3	item
1 pkg. medium flour tortilla	80-100	2	item
1 box bran flakes cereal	90-100	0	3/4c
1 bag french bread/rolls	70	1	item
reduced fat biscuit mix	1	.5	1/2c
8oz. lasagna noodles	1	2 oz	
1 bag whole wheat hamburger buns	15	1	2 oz
1 lb. medium barley	100	< 1	1 oz
1 pkg. manicotti shells	200	1	2 oz
5 lb. all purpose flour	400	1	1c
1 lb. whole wheat flour	350	2	1c
1 1/2 lb. spaghetti	210	1	1 oz

Meats

	Calorie	Fat	Serving
1 lb. turkey breast luncheon meat	60-70	1	2oz
4 lbs. chicken breast, boneless and skinless	130-150	2	3.5oz
3/4 lb. flank steak	207-218	11-12	3 oz
1 lb. fish- sole, flounder or cod	220-240	2	5 oz
3oz. boiled ham, 97% lean	37-45	1	1oz
1 1/2 lbs. fish- flounder, tiliapia, sole, cod, halibut, ocean perch, trout or orange roughy, fresh			
1 lb. snapper, fresh	93-100	1	3.5oz
3/4 lb ground sirloin	140	8	3 oz

Dairy

	Calorie	Fat	Serving

Serving

	Calorie	Fat	Serving
1/2 gal skim milk	90	0	1c

	Calorie	Fat	Serving
light strawberry cream cheese	60-80	5	1 oz
lite mayonnaise	35-50	1-5	1Tbsp
1 dozen eggs	79	5.6	1 med
2 lowfat yogurts	200	3-4	1c
1 qt. lowfat frozen yogurt	107-120	1	1/2c
1 pkg vanilla pudding	140	4	1/2c
1% cottage cheese	82-90	1	1/2c
1/2 lb. extra light margarine	45	0	2 Tbsp
fat free parmesan cheese	45	0	2Tbsp
8oz. light pizza cheese	70	4	1 oz
8oz. light cheddar cheese	70	4	1 oz
fat free sour cream	30	0	2Tbsp
8oz. lowfat mozzarella cheese	70	4	1 oz
fruit flavored sorbet	110-120	0-<1	4 oz

Miscellaneous
Rapid rise yeast
1/4 lb walnuts
1 can low sodium chicken broth
1 can regular chicken broth
1 can regular cream chicken soup
24oz. tomato sauce
6oz. tomato paste
2 14oz. cans stewed tomatoes
16oz, can pork and beans
2 14oz. no added fat pizza sauce
6oz. sliced black olives
2-3 bulbs fresh garlic
1 small jar salsa
1 bottle red wine
1 bottle white cooking wine
curry powder
nutmeg
cumin
garlic powder
thyme leaves
oregano, dried
onion powder

tarragon
basil leaves
cinnamon
red pepper
chili powder
paprika
salt
black pepper, whole
small bottle olive oil
small bottle canola oil
soy sauce
light ranch dressing
light salad dressing any variety
balsamic vinegar
12oz chili sauce
coarse grain dijon mustard
small bottle honey
spray vegetable oil
Sunbird stir fry seasoning
15oz. can black beans
15oz. can kidney beans
11oz. can corn
jelly any flavor
Decaf coffee or tea
diet sodas
bottled water if necessary, unflavored
Spike seasoning
Vegit seasoning

Week II

Fruit
2 bananas
1 apple any variety
2 oranges
1 small can pineapple in lite syrup
2 kiwi
1 small can tropical fruit
1 large can mandarin oranges
1 cantaloupe

Vegetables
1 head romaine lettuce
1 tomato
1 bunch fresh spinach
1 baker potato
2 new red potatoes
1 fresh bunch broccoli
2 yellow squash
1 small zucchini

Dairy
1/2 gal skim milk

The Recipes

Recipe 1

Chicken Salad Delight

3 cups	water
½ cup	medium barley
1 tsp.	Chicken bouillon
2 cups	chopped chicken breast
2 cups	halved seedless green or red grapes
½ cup	chopped celery
¼ cup	chopped walnuts
¾ cup	light mayonnaise
1 tbsp.	skim milk`
1 tsp.	curry powder (optional)

Bring water to a boil; stir in barley, bouillon granules and 1/4 tsp. salt. Reduce heat.   Cover; simmer 50-60 minutes or until tender, stirring occasionally. Drain; cool. Combine cooked barley, chicken grapes, celery and walnuts. Combine remaining 1/4 tsp. salt with remaining ingredients; mix well. Pour over barley mixture, tossing lightly. Cover, chill.

TIP: Serve in cantaloupe or on lettuce leaves. To reduce salt further omit the second 1/4 tsp.

Serves 7. Cals: 238 Cholesterol: 22mg. Fat: 6 gm. Sodium: 952 mg

Recipe 2

Manicotti

6-8	manicotti shells
1-1oz. pkg.	frozen chopped spinach
1/4 tsp.	ground nutmeg
12oz.	1% cottage cheese
2 tps.	chopped parsley
1	egg white
24oz.	tomato sauce
1/2 tsp	garlic powder
1/2 tsp	dried oregano
1/2 tsp.	dried basil
1/4-1/2 tsp.	white wine

Cook spinach with nutmeg in microwave as directed on package. Meanwhile, mash the cheese so it looks like a fine crumble. Beat the egg white with a fork until frothy; set aside. Squeeze all liquid out of cooked spinach. Add egg white , spinach , cheese and parsley. Mix thoroughly and set aside. Combine tomato sauce, garlic powder, oregano, basil, marjoram and wine in sauce pan. Cook over medium heat for several minutes. Stuff raw shells with filling. Place in pan with some sauce on bottom. Pour remaining sauce over shells. Cover and cook for 1 hour covered at 350.

Serves 8. Cals: 278 per shell Cholesterol: 44mg. Fat: 1 gm. Sodium: 1242 mg

Recipe 3

Chicken Pot Pie

2	large boneless, skinless chicken breast halves
2-16oz.	cans of mixed vegetables
1/4 cup	low sodium chicken broth
1 10 1/2 oz	can of cream of chicken soup
3/4 cup	skim milk
1 cup	reduced fat biscuit mix
1 tbsp.	Margarine

Cook chicken until done. Place in casserole dish. Add mixed vegetables that have been rinsed and drained. Add soup, and broth. Stir to mix well. In a separate bowl mix biscuit mix ,margarine and milk. Pour over casserole. Bake at 350 for 1 hour.

Serves 6. Cals: 365 Cholesterol: 24 mg. Fat: 13 gm Sodium 622 mg

Recipe 4
Oriental Oats Pilaf

1-1/2 cups	oats, uncooked
1	egg, beaten
1 cup	sliced white mushrooms
1/2 cup	sliced green onions
1/2 cup	celery
2 tsp.	Margarine
1/2 cup	chicken broth
2 tbsp.	Soysauce
2 tsp.	Sugar
6oz.	frozen pea pods, thawed

Combine oats and egg , mixing until oats are thoroughly coated. In medium skillet, saute mushrooms, green onions and celery in margarine 3 to 4 minutes or until tender. Add oat mixture; cook, stirring constantly, about 8 minutes or until oats are dry, separated and lightly browned. Add combined chicken broth, soy sauce and sugar; continue cooking 3 to5 minutes or until liquid is absorbed, stirring occasionally. Add pea pods; heat through.

Serves 6. Cals: 225 Cholesterol: 22mg. Fat: 2 gm. Sodium: 302 mg

Recipe 5

Beef Florentine

¾ lb.	lean flank steak
1 tsp.	canola oil
1 tbsp.	diced onions
10oz	frozen spinach
1 cup	water
1 med.	Tomato
1 tsp.	Salt
1 tsp.	Oregano
1 1/2 cup	brown rice, minute
1 tbsp.	Fat free parmesan cheese

Brown beef and onion in oil.. Push meat to side of pan and add spinach, water, tomato, salt and oregano. Break up spinach and bring to a boil. Stir in rice cover, remove form heat, and let stand 5 minutes. sprinkle with cheese and serve.

Serves 4. Cals: 280 Cholesterol: 22 mg. Fat: 7 Sodium: 661mg.

Notes:

Recipe 6

Garden Patch Salad

2 cups	water
1/3 cup	medium barley
3/4 tsp.	Salt
15 oz.	Canned light or red kidney beans, drained
3 med.	Tomatoes
1 1/2 cups	chopped parsley or cilantro fresh
1 med.	Green, red or yellow bell pepper, cut into strips
1/2 cup	sliced green onions
1/2 cup	light ranch dressing
1/8 tsp.	Cracked pepper

Bring water to a boil; stir in barley and 1/4tsp. salt. Reduce heat. Cover; simmer 50 to 60 minutes or until barley is tender, stirring occasionally. Drain; cool. Transfer to a large bowl. Add kidney beans, tomatoes, parsley, green pepper and green onions; mix well.
Combine lemon juice, oil, remaining 1/2 tsp. salt and pepper; mix until well blended. Pour over barley mixture; toss. Chill 3to 4 hours or over night; toss before serving.

Serves 8. Cals: 132 Cholesterol: 0 Fat: 4 gm. Sodium: 345 mg.

Recipe 7

Chicken Parmesan

4-4oz	skinless, boneless breast halves
1/2 tsp.	Pepper
1/2 cup	vegetable oil spray
1 tbsp.	Margarine
1/2 cup	sliced fresh white mushrooms
1 tbsp.	Sliced green onions
1 tbsp.	All-purpose flour
1 cup	skim milk
3 tbsp.	Fat free parmesan cheese
1/8 tsp.	Pepper

Brown chicken in a non stick skillet. Set chicken aside. In same skillet add margarine, mushrooms, and sliced green onions; saute until tender. Add flour; stir well. Gradually add milk; cook 1 minute or until thickened, stirring constantly. Add cheese and pepper; stir well. Add chicken and heat through. Serve over pasta or rice.

Serves 6. Cals: 197 Cholesterol: 4 mg. Fat: 9 gm. Sodium: 175 mg

Recipe 8

Cajun Baked Fish

2 tsp.	Canola oil
1 tbsp.	Paprika
2 tsp.	Thyme leaves, crushed
1 tsp.	Onion powder
1/2 tsp.	Garlic powder
1/4 tsp.	Salt
1/8-1/4 tsp.	Ground red pepper
1 lb.	fish fillets, sole, flounder or cod

Preheat oven to 400. In a small bowl combine oil, paprika, salt, and red pepper. Spread mixture evenly on one side of fish. Place fillets on a lightly greased pan seasoned side up. Bake until fish flakes about 8 to 10 minutes. Garnish with green pepper.

Serves 4. Cals:166 Cholesterol: 77mg. Fat: 4gm Sodium: 255 mg.

Recipe 9

Pizza

3 cups	all purpose flour
1 cup	whole wheat flour
1-1/2 cup	warm water`
1 tbsp.	Honey
1 small	purple onion, finely chopped
1 med.	green, yellow or red bell pepper, finely chopped
6oz.	white, cremini or portabella mushrooms, thinly sliced
6oz.	can sliced black olives
3oz.	chopped boiled ham
2-14oz.	jars of no-added fat pizza sauce
1-8oz.	pkg. light pizza cheese

Dilute yeast in warm water and honey. Let yeast activate. When foam appears the yeast is ready. Combine the rest of the ingredients. Add yeast slowly to flour so its evenly mixed. Mix until dough ball forms. Lightly spray bowl with cooking oil . Coat dough ball by rolling in bowl. Cover with plastic wrap and let rise; doubles in size. When dough is ready divide in half and roll out on floured surface. Form pizza crust. Top with the above ingredients. Bake at 450 for 20-25 minutes.

Serves 16. Cals: 208 per slice Cholesterol: 8mg. Fat: 5 gm Sodium: 367 mg.

Recipe 10

Chicken Stir Fry with Rice

2-4oz.	skinless, boneless chicken breast halves
14oz. Pkg.	frozen stir fry vegetables
1 pkg.	Sunbird stir fry seasoning mix
2 tbsp.	soy sauce
1 tsp.	Sugar
1/4 cup	water
1 cup	long grain brown rice, uncooked
2 cups	water
1/16 tsp.	Salt

Brown chicken breast in a little bit of water in wok. Add frozen vegetables, cook until tender. Mix stir fry seasoning according to package. Add to chicken and vegetable mixture. Mix rice , salt and water. Bring to a boil; simmer on low for 20 minutes or until rice is done. Serve stir fry over rice.

Serves 4. Cals: 121 Cholesterol 4 mg. Fat: 9 gm. Sodium: 70 mg.

Recipe 11

Brown Rice Black Bean Burrito

1 tbsp.	canola oil
1 med.	onion, chopped
2 cloves	garlic, minced
1 1/2 tsp.	chili powder
1/2 tsp.	Cumin
3 cups	cooked brown rice
15-16 oz.	canned black beans, drained and rinsed
11oz.	can corn, drained
6 - 8"	flour tortilla
3/4 cup (6oz.)	shredded reduced fat cheddar cheese
2	green onions, thinly sliced
1/4 cup	fat free sourcream
1/4 cup	salsa

Heat oil in large skillet over medium-high heat until hot. Add onion, garlic, chili powder and cumin. Saute 3-5 minutes until onion is tender. Add rice, beans and corn; cook stirring 2-3 minutes until mixture is thoroughly heated. Remove from heat. Spoon 1/2 cup rice mixture down center of each tortilla. Top each with 2 tbsp. of cheese, 1 tbsp. green onion and 1 tbsp. Sour cream; roll up top with salsa.

Serves 6. Cals: 466 Cholesterol: 11mg . Fat 5 gm Sodium: 604 mg

Recipe 12

Pasta Primavera

1 lb.1/2 pound	spaghetti
1 med.	Onion
2	cloves garlic
2 tsp.	Canola oil
4 med.	Tomatoes
1 med.	Zucchini
1 tsp.	Salt
1 tsp.	Basil, crushed
1/2-3/4 tsp.	Ground black pepper
1 lb.	Broccoli florets
1 cup	red wine
1/2 cup	chopped parsley
2 tbsp.	Tomato paste

Prepare spaghetti. Saute onion, garlic in oil until tender. Add tomatoes, zucchini, salt basil, and pepper. Stir 1 minute. Add broccoli and wine. Cover and simmer for 8 minutes. Stir parsley and tomato paste into sauce and cover over medium heat 1-2 minutes until it thickens. Serve over spaghetti.

Serves 8. Cals: 286 Cholesterol: 0 Fat: 3 gm Sodium: 346

Notes:

Recipe 13

Flounder Dijon

4	large carrots, julienned
2 tbsp.	parsley, minced
1 tps.	olive oil
1/8 tsp.	Salt
1/8 tsp.	Pepper
2 tsp.	coarse-grain dijon mustard
1 tsp.	Honey
4 (4-5oz.)	flounder, tilapia, sole, cod, catfish, halibut, ocean perch, roughy, or polluck

Combine carrots, parsley, salt and pepper in a 7x11x2 inch microwave safe dish. Cover with wax paper. Microwave at 100% power for 5 minutes. stirring once.

To make an even thickness, fold over thin fillets or bend long fillets. Place fillets on top of carrots in the corners of the dish with the thick parts toward the outside and the thin parts towards the center. Combine the mustard and honey and spread over fillets.
Cover with wax paper. Microwave at 100% power for 2 minutes. Rotate fillets, placing cooked parts toward the center and continue to cook for 1 to 3 minutes longer or just until fish flakes. Let stand, covered for 2 minutes.

Serves 4: Cals: 252 Cholesterol: 108 mg Fat: 4 gm. Sodium: 720 mg
TIP: To lower sodium leave out added salt.

Recipe 14

Seasoned Snapper

1 lb.	red snapper fillets
1 small	bottle fat free italian dressing
1/2 tsp.	cayenne pepper
1/2 tsp.	garlic, minced
1/2 tsp.	Tarragon
1/2 tsp.	minced parsley

Spray broiler pan with cooking spray. Coat the fillets in salad dressing. Mix seasonings and sprinkle over fish. Broil top rack for 3 to 4 minutes per side.

Serves 4. Cals: 118 Cholesterol: 41mg. Fat: 2gm Sodium; 175 mg

---

Notes:

Recipe 15

Lasagna

1 cup	chopped onion
3	cloves garlic
1 tsp.	canola oil
3/4 lb.	ground sirloin
2-14	stewed tomatoes
1/2 oz.	bottle chili sauce
6oz.	tomato paste
2 tsp.	dried basil leaves
1 tsp.	dried oregano leaves
1/2 tsp.	sugar (optional)
1/4 tsp.	Pepper
2 cups	nonfat cottage cheese
1/2 cup	1% grated parmesan cheese
1/4 cup	chopped parsley
8oz.	lasagna noodles
1 cup	shredded lowfat mozzarella cheese, divided

Saute onion and garlic in oil until tender. Push to one side of skillet. Add beef and brown. Add tomatoes, tomato paste, basil, oregano, sugar, and pepper. Simmer for 30 minutes. Combine cottage cheese, 1/4 cup parmesan cheese and parsley. Set aside. Layer meat sauce on bottom of pan , raw noodles, half of cottage cheese mixture, 2 tbsp. parmesan cheese, 1/3 cup mozzarella, and repeat. Bake at 350, 45 minutes covered with foil and bake an additional 15 minutes uncovered to brown.

Serve 12. Cals: 266 Cholesterol: 27mgs Fat: 6gm. Sodium: 513 mg

Recipe 16

Sloppy Bean Joes

1/2 pound	ground sirloin
1/2 cup	chopped green bell pepper
1/2 cup	chopped onion
16 oz.	Canned pork and beans
12 oz.	Bottle chili sauce
8	whole wheat hamburger buns

Brown ground beef with green pepper and onion; drain. Add remaining ingredients except buns; simmer for 5-10 minutes or until heated through. Toast buns. Arrange buns halves on plate, pour been mixture on top.

Serves 8. Cals: 255 Cholesterol: 22 mg Fat: 6 gm. Sodium: 952 mg

Recipe 17

Pasta with Spinach Sauce

1 lb.1/2 pound	fresh spinach
1 lb.	Lowfat ricotta cheese
2	egg whites
2	cloves garlic, minced
1/2 cup	grated fat free parmesan cheese
1/2 tsp.	Grated nutmeg
1 lb.	Spaghetti, raw

Remove the stems from spinach. Wash, drain and dry. Put spinach in food processor; process. Add ricotta, egg, garlic, cheese and nutmeg. Mix at high speed. Set sauce aside. Prepare spaghetti. Drain. Toss sauce with pasta and cook through.

Serves 8. Cals:286 Cholesterol: 0 Fat:3 gm. Sodium: 346mgs

Day 1

Breakfast	**Lunch**	**Dinner**
1 Raisin cinnamon bagel	Chicken Salad Delight**	Manicotti**
1 T light cream cheese	½ cup cantaloupe	1 cup romaine salad
1/2 cup cinnamon	5 whole wheat crackers	Balsamic vinegar
applesauce	1 cup water	1 oz french bread/roll
1 cup decaf coffee or tea	12 oz diet soda	4oz red wine
1 cup water		

Cals: 252	Cals: 344	Cals: 503
Chol: 9mg	Chol: 22mg	Chol: 44mg
Fat 2.3 gm.	Fat: 9 gm	Fat: 2.5 gm
Sodium: 311 mg	Sodium: 1156mg	Sodium: 1506 mg

**Daily total: Calories: 1099   Cholesterol: 75 mg Fat :14 gm
Sodium: 2973 mg**

Day 2

Breakfast	**Lunch**	**Dinner**
2 frozen pancakes	Turkey sandwich	Chicken pot pie**
2 tbsp. apple butter	1 oz turkey breast	1 cup steamed spinach
1/2 cup peaches 1 tbsp lite mayo		1 x 1oz wheat roll
1 cup decaf coffee/tea	2 sls whole wheat brd	½ cup apricots
1 cup water	½ cup raw baby carrots	1 cup water
	1 apple	
	1 cup water	
	12 oz diet soda	

Cals: 316	Cals: 312	Cals: 595
Chol: 3mg	Chol: 21 mg	Chol: 24 mg
Fat: 14 gm	Fat: 7 gm	Fat: 14 gm
Sodium: 778 mg	Sodium: 804 mg	Sodium: 1028

**Daily Totals Calories: 1223 Cholesterol: 48mg   Fat: 22gm
Sodium: 2610mg**

**indicates recipe provided in this program

Day 3

Breakfast	Lunch	Dinner
2 Lite Blueberry Muffins	Oriental Oats Pilaf**	Beef Florentine**
1/2 cup cantaloupe	1 cup red grapes	1 cup brown rice
1 cup decaf coffee /tea	1 cup steamed broccoli	1 whole broiled tomato
1 cup water	1 cup water	with basil
1 cup water	12 oz diet soda	½ cup tropical fruit

Cals: 173	Cals: 394	Cals: 632
Chol: 0mg	Chol: 22 mg	Chol; 22mg
Fat: 2 gm	Fat: 3 gm	Fat: 9 gm
Sodium: 289 mg	Sodium: 378 mg	Sodium: 691 mg

**Daily Totals: Calories: 1199   Cholesterol: 44 mg   Fat: 14 gm
Sodium: 1358 mg**

Day 4

Breakfast	Lunch	Dinner
Vegetable omelet w/ 1 egg	Garden patch salad**	Chicken Parmesan**
1 oat bran english muffin	½ cup peach halves	1 cup tricolor pasta
2 tsp. Jelly	1 x 1oz whole wheat roll	1 cup steamd grn beans
1/2 pink grapefruit	1 cup water	1 cup grapes
1 cup decaf coffee or tea	12 oz diet soda	1 cup decaf coffee/tea
1 cup water		1 cup water

Cals: 329	Cals: 265	Cals: 562
Chol: 392 mg	Chol: 0	Chol: 180 mg
Fat: 14 gm	Fat: 5 gm	Fat: 13 gm
Sodium: 519 mg	Sodium: 539 mg	Sodium: 227 mg

**Daily Totals: Calories: 1156   Cholesterol: 572 mg   Fat: 32 gm
Sodium: 1285 mg**

Day 5

Breakfast	**Lunch**	**Dinner**
6-8oz. Lowfat yogurt	Cajun baked fish**	Pizza**
2 tbsp. grape nuts	1 cup wild rice	1 cup romaine salad
1 apple any variety	1 cup steamed carrots	Balsamic vinegar
1 cup decaf coffee or tea	½ cup apricots	1x1oz frenchbread/roll
1 cup water	1 cup water	½ cup pineapple
	12 oz diet soda	1 cup water

Cals: 318	Cals: 523	Cals: 611
Chol: 5 mg	Chol: 77 mg	Chol: 8 mg
Fat: 1 gm	Fat: 5 gm	Fat: 7gm
Sodium: 241 mg	Sodium: 452 mg	Sodium: 621 mg

**Daily Totals: Calories: 1452   Cholesterol: 90 mg   Fat: 13 gm
Sodium: 1314 mg**

Day 6

Breakfast	**Lunch**	**Dinner**
2 frozen waffles	Chicken Stir fry**	Rice/BeanBurrito*
2 tbsp. lite syrup	1 cup brown rice	1 cup steamed yellow
1/2 cup tropical fruit	1 cup Romaine salad	squash w/red peppers
1 cup decaf coffee or tea	balsamic vinegar	1 cup water
1 cup water	½ cup pineapple	12oz lite beer(optional)
	1 cup water	

Cals: 332	Cals: 418	Cals: 502
Chol: 0	Chol: 3 mg	Chol: 11 mg
Fat: 7 gm	Fat: 11 gm	Fat: 6 gm
Sodium: 623 mg	Sodium: 153 mg	Sodium: 613 mg

**Daily Totals: Calories: 1253   Cholesterol: 14 mg   Fat: 24 gm
Sodium: 1389 mg**

Day 7

Breakfast	Lunch	Dinner
1 cup bran flakes	Pasta Primavera**	Flounder Dijon**
1 cup skim milk	1 ½ cups	1 cup brown rice
1/2 pink grapefruit	1x1oz french bread/roll	1 cup mix vegetables
1 cup decaf coffee/tea	½ cup tropical fruit	1 cup water
1 cup water	1 cup water	1 cup decaf coffee/tea
	12 oz diet soda	
Cals: 390	Cals: 498	Cals: 581
Chol: 4 mg	Chol: 0	Chol: 108mg
Fat: 2 gm	Fat: 4 gm	Fat: 6 gm
Sodium: 502 mg	Sodium: 570 mg	Sodium: 797 mg

**Daily Totals: Calories: 1469   Cholesterol: 112 mg   Fat: 12gm
Sodium: 1869 mg**

Day 8

Breakfast	Lunch	Dinner
1 oat bran english muffin	Turkey sandwich	Pizza (2 slices)**
4oz. lowfat yogurt	1oz turkey breast	1 cup Romaine salad
1 Tbsp. Xtra lite marg.or	1 tbsp lite mayo	Balsamic vinegar
2tsp jelly	lettuce and tomato	1x1oz french bread/roll
1 jr. Banana	2 slices whole wheat bread	½ cup sorbet
1 cup decaf coffee/tea	1 apple	
	1 cup water	
	12 oz diet soda	
Cals: 40	Cals: 280	Cals: 631
Chol: 5 mg	Chol: 26 mg	Chol: 8mg
Fat: 8 gm	Fat: 7 gm	Fat: 9 gm
Sodium: 348 mg	Sodium: 703 mg	Sodium: 654 mg

**Daily Total: Calories: 1318 Cholesterol: 39 mg   Fat: 24 gm
Sodium:1705 mg**

Day 9

Breakfast	Lunch	Dinner
1 cup bran flakes	Spinach Salad	Beef Florentine**
1 cup skim milk	2 oz Turkey breast	1 cup brown rice
1 slice whole wheat toast	1 chopped egg	1x1oz whole wheat roll
1 tbp. xtra lite marg.	½ cup sliced mushrooms	½ cup frozen yogurt
or 2 tsp. Jelly	2 tbsp lite dressing	1 cup water
1 cup decaf coffee or tea	5 whole wheat crackers	
1 cup water	1 orange	
	1 cup water	
	12 oz diet soda	
Cals: 463	Cals:329	Cals: 793
Chol: 4 mg	Chol: 165 mg	Chol: 24 mg
Fat: 5 gm	Fat: 12 gm	Fat: 9 gm
Sodium: 668 mg	Sodium: 1163 mg	Sodium: 1004 mg

**Daily Totals: Calories: 1585   Cholesterol: 193 mg   Fat: 31 gm
Sodium: 2835**

Day 10

Breakfast	Lunch	Dinner
2 frozen waffles	Lasagna**	3oz chopped sirloin
1 Tbsp. lite syrup	1 cup Romaine salad	1 cup steamed carrots
1/2 cup sliced strawberries	1 tbsp lite dressing	1 med baked potato
1 cup milk	1 orange	1 tbsp xtra lite marg
1 cup decaf coffee or tea	1 cup water	½ cup pineapple
	12 oz diet soda	1 cup water
Cals: 368	Cals: 134	Cals 531
Chol: 4 mg	Chol: 27 mg	Chol: 76 mg
Fat: 8 gm	Fat: 9 gm	Fat: 12 gm
Sodium: 743 mg	Sodium: 710 mg	Sodium: 186 mg

**Daily Totals: Calories: 1033 Cholesterol: 107 mg   Fat: 29 gm
Sodium: 1639 mg**

Day 11

Breakfast	**Lunch**	**Dinner**
1 egg scrambled	Sloppy Bean Joes**	Seasoned Snapper**
2 whole wheat toast	1 cup steamed yellow	2 steamed new potatoes
2 tsp. Jelly	squash w/ucchini	1 cup steamed broccoli
1 kiwi sliced	1 Tbsp lite ranch dressing	½ cup vanilla pudding
1 cup decaf coffee or tea	½ cup tropical fruit	1 cup water
1 cup water	12 oz diet soda	
Cals: 325	Cals: 356	Cals: 467
Chol: 399 mg	Chol; 22 mg	Chol: 42 mg
Fat: 12 gm	Fat: 7 gm	Fat: 4 gm
Sodium: 633 mg	Sodium: 984 mg	Sodium: 285 mg

Daily Totals: Calories:1148　　　**Cholesterol: 463 mg**　　　**Fat:23 gm**
Sodium:1902 mg

Day 12

Breakfast	**Lunch**	**Dinner**
2 frozen pancakes	Turkey sandwich	Cajun fish**
2 Tbsp. lite syrup	2 oz turkey breast	1 cup wild rice
1/2 cup cantaloupe	1 tbsp lite mayo	1 cup steamed broccoli
1 cup skim milk	lettuce and tomato	
1 cup decaf coffee/tea	2 slices whole wheat bread	
1 cup water	½ cup mandarin oranges	
	1 cup water	
Cals: 184	Cals: 280	Cals: 383
Chol: 4 mg	Chol: 26 mg	Chol: 77 mg
Fat: 1 gm	Fat: 7 gm	Fat: 5 gm
Sodium: 517 mg	Sodium: 703 mg	Sodium: 312 mg

Daily Totals: Calories: 847　　　**Cholesterol: 107 mg**　　　**Fat: 13 gm**
Sodium: 1532 mg

Day 13

Breakfast	**Lunch**	**Dinner**
2 whole wheat toast	Chicken Salad delight**	Manicotti**
2 tsp. Jelly	½ cup cantaloupe	1x1oz french bread/roll
6oz. lowfat yogurt	5 whole wheat crackers	Balsamic vinegar
1 jr. Banana	1 cup water	1 cup water
1 cup decaf coffee or tea	12 oz diet soda	
1 cup water		
Cals: 308	Cals: 344	Cals: 503
Chol: 5 mg	Chol: 22 mg	Chol: 44 mg
Fat: 3 gm	Fat: 9 gm	Fat: 2.5 gm
Sodium: 420 mg	Sodium: 1156	Sodium: 1506

**Daily Totals: Calories: 1155   Cholesterol: 71 mg   Fat: 14.5 gm
Sodium: 3082**

Day 14

Breakfast	**Lunch**	**Dinner**
6-8 oz Low fat yogurt	Garden patch salad**	Chicken Parmesan**
2 tbsp grape nuts	½ cup peach halves	1 cup tricolor pasta
1 apple	1x1oz whole wheat roll	1 cup steamed green
1 cup decaf coffee/tea	1 cup water	beans
1 cup water	12 oz diet soda	1 cup water
Cals: 318	Cals: 265	Cals: 562
Chol: 5 mg	Chol: 0	Chol: 180 mg
Fat: 1 gm	Fat: 5 gm	Fat: 13 gm
Sodium: 241 mg	Sodium: 539 mg	Sodium: 227 mg

**Daily Totals: Calories: 1145   Cholesterol: 185 mg   Fat: 19 gm
Sodium: 1007 mg**

Snacks

The following are suggestion for snacks. The caloric intake for the day determines whether a snack is allowed. As you look over the menu you will notice the calorie level varies from day to day. That is because some meals are heavier than others.

You may choose a snack based on the calorie level and your allowance for that day. It is not recommended to replace your meal plan with snacks because the menu is nutritionally balanced. You should look at snacks as a compliment to your meal plan.

The following is a generalized list of recommended foods so you can choose and buy appropriately. Note fat free treats are not necessary because fat was saved in the menu to allow for this. Reduced fat snacks are also acceptable.

Serving	Calories	Fat
Lowfat frozen yogurt (1/2 cup)	120	1
Lowfat icecream (1/2 cup)	120	4
Fruit sorbet (1/2) cup	110-120	0
Frozen fruit juice bars (1 bar)	70-90	0-3
Reduced fat cookies/crackers (any variety) (2-5)	60-80	2
Reduced fat chips, potato, or corn . (< 1oz.)	130-150	6
Pretzels (1 oz.)	110	1
Mini bagels (2)	70-90	1
Vanilla wafers *0)	185	7

Graham crackers, any flavor (2)	60	1
Ginger snap cookies (0.5 oz)	64	2
Angelfood cake (1/12)	130-150	0
Cereals any variety (1 oz)	90-180	2
Fresh fruit (1 piece)	40-80	0
Dried fruit (1 oz)	90-150	1
Nutrigrain bar (1 bar)	130-150	3
Granola bars (1 bar)	100-140	1-3

**For chocoholics:
Reduced fat chocolate sandwich cookies
Lowfat chocolate flavored yogurt, in refrigerated section of store.
Lowfat chocolate icecream.

Note serving size is on label. This is the allowed portion.
The above nutritional Information is an average.

The DINING OUT guide

In this guide you will find general advice about dining-out as well as tips on eating in specific ethnic restaurants.

<u>General Tips</u>

♦ Decide what you are going to have ahead of time

♦ Don't go hungry

♦ Have a glass of water or diet soda

♦ Order a salad

♦ Have salad dressing and sauces on the side

♦ Dip fork into salad dressing then into salad, not vice-versa

♦ Specify small portions/choose appetizer size/split entrees

♦ Be assertive

♦ Focus on the conversation

♦ Ask for leftover food to be cleared away quickly

♦ Do not take doggie bags

♦ Watch the desserts! Choose coffee or cappuccino with skim milk

♦ Avoid the bread and chips

♦ Wear tight clothes

♦ Go with supportive friends

CHINESE

SELF-ESTEEM ENHANCERS

Soups
Tofu (Bean curd)
Lobster sauce
Assorted vegetables
White rice
Lo Mein with vegetables
"steamed"
"stir fried"
"roasted"
"simmered"

HEALTH BUSTERS

Egg rolls	Soy sauce
Spring rolls	Plum sauce
Fried rice	Hoisin sauce
Sweet and Sour	MSG
Cashews	
Peanuts	

"fried"
"crispy"
"battered"

Ask: Food to be prepared in as little oil as possible
Food to be prepared without MSG and Salt
Leave out the nuts
Remove crispy fried noodles

Tip: *Fortune cookie say " A healthy eater is one who takes fortune to heart but leaves cookie on table."*
****

ITALIAN

SELF-ESTEEM ENHANCERS

Marinara sauce
Cacciatore
Light sauces
Florentine
Grilled
Clam sauce
Primavera (no cream)
Piccata
Chicken   Fish

HEALTH BUSTERS

Alfredo   Cream sauce
Parmigiana   Veal
Carbonara   Calamari
Prosciutto
Cheese
Manicotti
Sausage
Cannelloni

Ask: Sauce on the side
Salad dressing on the side
Hold the Parmesan cheese and pine nuts
Remove the bread
Where is the nearest drycleaner?

Tip: *Watch out for the desserts! Order plain coffee or capuccino made with skimmed milk. Or else lock yourself in the bathroom while the others are eating.*

MEXICAN

SELF-ESTEEM ENHANCERS	HEALTH BUSTERS	
Chicken	Nachos	Quesadillas
Salsa	Cheese	Chorizo
Salsa verde	Guacamole	Sopaipillas
Enchilada sauce	Chimichanga	
Tortilla (no cheese, sour cream)	Flauta	
Picante sauce	Chile relleno	
Enchilada (no sour cream, cheese)	Sour cream	
Chili con carne (no cheese, sour cream)	Corn chips	
Fajitas (no cheese, sour cream, guacamole)	Chili con queso	
Black beans	Refried beans	
Mexican rice	Fried tortilla shells	

Ask: Remove/minimize the sour cream, cheese, guacamole and chips
Salsa as salad dressing

Tip: *Avoid the combination plates and stick to just one Margarita.*
****

THAI

SELF-ESTEEM ENHANCERS	HEALTH BUSTERS
Tom Yum Koong	Tod Mun
Pla Koong	Tom Ka Gai
Yam Yai	Crispy Duck
Thai Chicken	Praram long song
Sweet and Sour Chicken	Hot Thai Catfish
Chili Duck	Spareribs curry
"Thai spices"	"Peanut sauce"
"braised"	"coconut milk"
"chili sauce"	"golden brown duck"

Ask: Preparation in vegetable oil as opposed to coconut
Hold the MSG
Leave out the nuts
Reduce the salt and soy content
Do I need a coat and Thai?

Tip: *Eat the steamed white rice and go for as much spiciness as you wish.*

INDIAN

SELF-ESTEEM ENHANCERS
Papadum
Nan
Mulligatawny
Chicken Tandoori
Chicken Tikka
"biryani"
"pullao"
"raita"
"mango chutney"

HEALTH BUSTERS
Samosa
Paratha or Poori
Coconut soup
Shrimp curry
Chicken Kandhari
"curry"
"masala"
"ghee"
"Koulfi"

Ask: For plenty of water
Minimize the dried fruits
For the plain rice
For hot tea with the main meal

Tip: *Vegetables and spices dominate Indian food so it's relatively easy to find healthy, low-fat meals. Just watch out for the sauces.*
****

JAPANESE

SELF-ESTEEM ENHANCERS
Sashimi
Sushi
Yakitori
Sukiyaki
"broiled" (yaki)
"steamed" (mushimono)
"grilled" (yakimono)
"seasoned rice"

HEALTH BUSTERS
Tempura
Agemono
Katsu

"fried"
"battered"

Ask: How fresh is the sushi?
Tone down the soy
Which one is the wasabe?
How do you cut it that fast?

Tip: *Japanese food is generally very healthy and low in fat. Just watch some of the sauces and avoid the fried stuff and you'll be okay*

FRENCH

SELF-ESTEEM ENHANCERS	**HEALTH BUSTERS**
Gazpacho	French Onion Soup
Shrimp	Pate
Petite filet mignon	Escargots
Lamb	Steak
"grilled" (grille)	"au gratin"
"fruit sauces"	"en croute"
"en brochette"	"cream sauce"
"petite"	"casserole"

Ask: Put the sauce on the side
      Leave off the sour cream
      Don't bring the croissants or dinner rolls
      Leave the butter in the kitchen
      What wine would you recommend?

Tip: Be careful a la French restaurant. The food can be tres rich and there can be beaucoup de fat.

****

PIZZA

SELF-ESTEEM ENHANCERS	**HEALTHBUSTERS**
Crust	Bacon
Green/red peppers	Prosciutto (ham)
Mushrooms	Meatballs
Pineapple	Sausage
Eggplant	Anchovies
Onions	Pepperoni
Olives	Extra cheese
Chicken	

Ask: How big are the slices?
      Not too much cheese
      Split the toppings
      Am I right in assuming that this is the owner's grandmother's very own
      special recipe?

Tip: *Pizza can be a very acceptable healthy food if you minimize the cheese, choose healthier toppings and do not eat too many slices.*

THE SALAD BAR

SELF-ESTEEM ENHANCERS
Low fat Blue Cheese Dressing
Vinegar
Non-Oil dressings
Reduced calorie Blue cheese dressing
Reduced calorie Russian dressing
Raisins
Chinese noodles
Fruit
Cottage cheese
Tuna

HEALTHBUSTERS
All regular dressings
Reduced calorie Italian dressing
Reduced calorie Thousand Island
Reduced calorie French
Mayonnaise
Sesame seeds
Peanuts
Bacon bits
Pepperoni
Potato salad

Ask: What is this salad marinated in?
Is there Mayo in this salad?
What's in the House dressing?
How many trips to the salad bar do I get?

Tip: *Salad dressing is the greatest source of fat for many women. Always have the dressing served on the side and dip your fork into the salad dressing first, then into the salad. You end up eating about 10% of the dressing and still get the taste.*
****

SEAFOOD

SELF-ESTEEM ENHANCERS
Broiled
Blackened
Barbecued
Steamed
Stir fried

HEALTHBUSTERS
Fried
Breaded
Battered
Baked
Fish and Chips (really Fries)
Chowder
Bisque   Creamy

Ask: How is the fish prepared?
What's in the sauce?
Sauce on the side?
What's the portion size?
Can I split the entree?

Tip: *Most fish is a good healthy choice so don't ruin it by adulterating it with fat toppings and sauces.*

FAST FOOD

SELF-ESTEEM ENHANCERS

Salad
Baked potato
Single plain hamburger
Grilled chicken sandwich
Non-fried fish sandwich

Low-fat yogurt
Juice

HEALTHBUSTERS

Cheeseburgers
Oversized burgers
Fried chicken
Chicken sandwich with cheese
Nugget style chicken
French fries
Onion rings
Milk shake

Ask: For a kids meal
         For reduced calorie dressing
         May I have some water?

Tip: *If you're having a salad watch out for the dressing? Also, don't eat it too fast. The average time to consume a typical fast food meal (over a thousand calories) is less than five minutes*
****

ALCOHOL

SELF-ESTEEM ENHANCERS

Light beer
Spritzers with diet mixer
Sweet drinks made with distilled spirits

HEALTHBUSTERS

Beer
Wine
Brandy, Kalhua, Amaretto, etc
Specialty drinks with whipped cream

The main concerns with alcohol are:

- The number of calories, particularly in the liqueurs and spirits where there can be up to 150 calories per shot
- The calories are essentially empty calories, i.e. have little nutritional value
- Alcohol stimulates the appetite for many people
- Willpower dissolves in alcohol
- Self-awareness and judgement also dissolve in alcohol
- After about five ounces of alcohol you are more likely to store fat

Tip: *Enjoy drinking in moderation - a glass of wine once in a while. Be careful, alcohol has the potential to be a very subtle dietbuster.*

MISCELLANEOUS AMERICAN STYLE

SELF-ESTEEM ENHANCERS

Peel and Eat shrimp
Chili
Cajun chicken sandwich
Stir fry
Fajitas (sauce on side)
Gyros
Shish kebab
Rice
Baked potato

Sorbet
Low-fat yogurt

HEALTHBUSTERS

Mozzarella sticks
Potato skins
Buffalo wings
Philly cheese steak
Ribs
Coleslaw (with mucho Mayo)
Quiche
Fries

Mud Pie
Ice cream
Cheesecake

Ask: For small portions
        For a glass of water
        How is this made?

Tip: *Keep track and minimize the fat wherever possible.*

****

NOTES:

The Personal HealthScope

The Personal HealthScope is designed to keep you focused on your goals and to help you keep rack of important behaviors. Each day includes a place to write your goals, a place to check off your actual behavior and reminders about the keys to success.

GOALS: These are listed under the category "Things I Want To Do Today."

EATING: Enter the number representing the upper limit of your desired calorie intake for the day. Do the same for fat grams

Circle the "No Bingeing" label if you intend to avoid bingeing. Do the same for "No Alcohol" if you intend to have an alcohol-free day.

EXERCISES: Circle the "Aerobics" label if you did an aerobic-type exercise. Do the same for "Stretching" and "Resistance."

ACTUAL BEHAVIOR: Circle the labels for those behaviors you actually did today.

CALCULATIONS: Record the calories and fat grams consumed at each meal and in snacks.

CONGRATULATIONS: Write down any behaviors you were pleased with today.

CONFESSIONS: Write down were you deviated significantly from your goals.

You will see that there is a weekly meeting with yourself every seventh day. During that meeting complete the page by circling the appropriate labels.

Personal HealthScope
        Date_____

Things I Want To Do Today

Eat no more than _____ calories   Avoid
Bingeing

Eat no more than _____ fat grams   Avoid alcohol

Calculations:

                           Breakfast   Lunch   Dinner   Snacks
Calories

Fat grams

Things I Did Today

Ate ___ calories   Ate _____ fat grams   Did not binge

Did not drink alcohol

Aerobic exercise   Stretching   Resistance   Imagery

Congratulations:

Confessions:

Considerations: Every action you take is your choice

Personal HealthScope   Date_____

Things I Want To Do Today

Eat no more than _____ calories   Avoid Bingeing

Eat no more than _____ fat grams   Avoid alcohol

Calculations:

	Breakfast	Lunch	Dinner	Snacks
Calories				
Fat grams				

Things I Did Today

Ate ___ calories   Ate _____ fat grams   Did not binge

Did not drink alcohol

Aerobic exercise   Stretching   Resistance   Imagery

Congratulations:

Confessions:

Considerations: The journey of a thousand miles begins with putting your sneakers on

Personal HealthScope　　　　　　　**Date**_____

Things I Want To Do Today

Eat no more than _____ calories　　　　　Avoid Bingeing

Eat no more than _____ fat grams　　　　Avoid alcohol

Calculations:

	Breakfast	Lunch	Dinner	Snacks
Calories				
Fat grams				

Things I Did Today

Ate ____ calories　　　　　Ate _____ fat grams　　Did not binge

Did not drink alcohol

Aerobic exercise　　　Stretching　　　Resistance　　　Imagery

Congratulations:

Confessions:

Considerations: Serving others requires taking care of yourself

Personal HealthScope   Date_____

Things I Want To Do Today

Eat no more than ____ calories   Avoid Bingeing

Eat no more than _____ fat grams   Avoid alcohol

Calculations:

	Breakfast	Lunch	Dinner	Snacks
Calories				
Fat grams				

Things I Did Today

Ate ___ calories   Ate ____ fat grams   Did not binge

Did not drink alcohol

Aerobic exercise   Stretching   Resistance   Imagery

Congratulations:

Confessions:

Considerations: This is the first day of the rest of your strife

Personal HealthScope   Date_____

Things I Want To Do Today

Eat no more than _____ calories   Avoid Bingeing

Eat no more than _____ fat grams   Avoid alcohol

Calculations:

	Breakfast	Lunch	Dinner	Snacks
Calories				
Fat grams				

Things I Did Today

Ate ___ calories   Ate _____ fat grams   Did not binge

Did not drink alcohol

Aerobic exercise   Stretching   Resistance   Imagery

Congratulations:

Confessions:

Considerations: You're not an egg so don't beat yourself up

Personal HealthScope　　　　　　　**Date**_____

Things I Want To Do Today

Eat no more than _____ calories　　　　　Avoid Bingeing

Eat no more than _____ fat grams　　　　Avoid alcohol

Calculations:

	Breakfast	Lunch	Dinner	Snacks
Calories				
Fat grams				

Things I Did Today

Ate ____ calories　　　　　Ate _____ fat grams　　Did not binge

Did not drink alcohol

Aerobic exercise　　　Stretching　　　Resistance　　　Imagery

Congratulations:

Confessions:

Considerations: Accept nothing except your humanity

Personal HealthScope   **Date**_____

Things I Want To Do Today

Eat no more than ____ calories   Avoid Bingeing

Eat no more than ___ __ fat grams   Avoid alcohol

Calculations:

	Breakfast	Lunch	Dinner	Snacks
Calories				
Fat grams				

Things I Did Today

Ate ___ calories   Ate ___ _ fat grams   Did not binge

Did not drink alcohol

Aerobic exercise   Stretching   Resistance   Imagery

Congratulations:

Confessions:

Considerations: What has happened to you before is history. Don't confuse the *historical* you with the *real* you.

WEEKLY REVIEW

Circle the labels that represent your behavior for the week

Took time for myself   Had appropriate boundaries
Stayed focused   Flushed away toxic thoughts
Respected my body   Communicated effectively

Overall in the past week I met my eating, exercise and self-care goals:
(*Circle the appropriate percentage*)

100%   80%   60%   40%   20%
0%

If you met your goals to at least the 60% level give yourself a reward.

My reward is _____

This week I need to watch out for the following situations:
....
....
....
I am going to cope by:
....
....
....

Now set your eating, exercise and self-care goals for the upcoming week

Personal HealthScope　　　　　　　**Date**_____

Things I Want To Do Today

Eat no more than _____ calories　　　　　　Avoid Bingeing

Eat no more than _____ fat grams　　　　Avoid alcohol

Calculations:

	Breakfast	Lunch	Dinner	Snacks
Calories				
Fat grams				

Things I Did Today

Ate ____ calories　　　　　Ate _____ fat grams　　Did not binge

Did not drink alcohol

Aerobic exercise　　　Stretching　　　Resistance　　　Imagery

Congratulations:

Confessions:

Considerations: People change when they experience a conflict in values, when there is too much disparity between their actions and their beliefs

Personal HealthScope   **Date**_____

Things I Want To Do Today

Eat no more than _____ calories   Avoid Bingeing

Eat no more than _____ fat grams   Avoid alcohol

Calculations:

                              Breakfast   Lunch Dinner Snacks

Calories

Fat grams

Things I Did Today

Ate ____ calories   Ate _____ fat grams   Didn't binge

Didn't drink alcohol

Aerobic exercise   Stretching   Resistance   Imagery

Congratulations:

Confessions:

Considerations: You can't take care of yourself if you're running on empty

Personal HealthScope   Date_____

Things I Want To Do Today

Eat no more than _____ calories   Avoid Bingeing

Eat no more than _____ fat grams   Avoid alcohol

Calculations:

	Breakfast	Lunch	Dinner	Snacks
Calories				
Fat grams				

Things I Did Today

Ate ___ calories   Ate ____ fat grams   Did not binge

Did not drink alcohol

Aerobic exercise   Stretching   Resistance   Imagery

Congratulations:

Confessions:

Considerations: We are social animals. There is nothing greater than making meaningful contact with another human being

Personal HealthScope   Date_____

Things I Want To Do Today

Eat no more than _____ calories   Avoid Bingeing

Eat no more than _____ fat grams   Avoid alcohol

Calculations:

	Breakfast	Lunch	Dinner	Snacks
Calories				
Fat grams				

Things I Did Today

Ate ___ calories   Ate _____ fat grams   Did not binge

Did not drink alcohol

Aerobic exercise   Stretching   Resistance   Imagery

Congratulations:

Confessions:

**Considerations: We are not smart enough to know all of the
risks inherent in our lifestyle. We should at least be smart
enough to avoid the risks we do know**

Personal HealthScope   Date_____

Things I Want To Do Today

Eat no more than ____ calories   Avoid Bingeing

Eat no more than _____ fat grams   Avoid alcohol

Calculations:

	Breakfast	Lunch	Dinner	Snacks
Calories				
Fat grams				

Things I Did Today

Ate ___ calories   Ate ____ fat grams   Did not binge

Did not drink alcohol

Aerobic exercise   Stretching   Resistance   Imagery

Congratulations:

Confessions:

Considerations: When working out, don't use your mind to time your exercise, use the time to exercise your mind.

Personal HealthScope   Date_____

Things I Want To Do Today

Eat no more than _____ calories   Avoid Bingeing

Eat no more than _____ fat grams   Avoid alcohol

Calculations:

	Breakfast	Lunch	Dinner	Snacks
Calories				
Fat grams				

Things I Did Today

Ate ___ calories   Ate _____ fat grams   Did not binge

Did not drink alcohol

Aerobic exercise   Stretching   Resistance   Imagery

Congratulations:

Confessions:

Considerations: Exercise is an appointment with yourself you have to keep.

Personal HealthScope Date_____

Things I Want To Do Today

Eat no more than _____ calories   Avoid Bingeing

Eat no more than _____ fat grams   Avoid alcohol

Calculations:

	Breakfast	Lunch	Dinner	Snacks
Calories				
Fat grams				

Things I Did Today

Ate ___ calories   Ate _____ fat grams   Did not binge

Did not drink alcohol

Aerobic exercise   Stretching   Resistance   Imagery

Congratulations:

Confessions:

Considerations: Do not let the restaurant owner, the chef or the server determine how much you're going to eat - they don't pay your medical bills

WEEKLY REVIEW

Circle the labels that represent your behavior for the week

Took time for myself   Had appropriate boundaries
Stayed focused   Flushed away toxic thoughts
Respected my body   Communicated effectively

Overall in the past week I met my eating, exercise and self-care goals:
(*Circle the appropriate percentage*)

100%   80%   60%   40%   20%
0%

If you met your goals to at least the 60% level give yourself a reward.

My reward is _____

This week I need to watch out for the following situations:
....
....
....

I am going to cope by:
....
....
....

Now set your eating, exercise and self-care goals for the upcoming week

INDEX

About the Authors

Howard J. Rankin Ph.D is a licensed clinical psychologist and expert on compulsive behaviors with an international reputation in the areas of wellness, eating disorders and lifestyle change. He has published over fifty scientific papers and has edited several prestigious journals. He was Chief of The Eating Disorders Unit, St. Andrews Hospital, Northampton, England and researcher at the Addiction Research Unit, at the Institute of Psychiatry in London. He has held academic positions at the University of London, where he obtained both his masters and doctoral degrees in clinical psychology and at the University of South Carolina where he is currently adjunct professor in the School of Public Health.

Dr. Rankin has written regularly for the mass market and was a regular contributor to the European version of Psychology Today. He is also the author of the book, "10 Steps to a Great Relationship; What every couple should know about love (Stepwise, 1998)

In addition to his writing, Dr Rankin is the executive director and founder of the Carolina Wellness Retreat, a lifestyle change program located on Hilton Head Island and at other locations throughout the Carolinas. For more information for Dr. Rankin's professional activities, including his seminars and workshops, please visit his website at www.howardrankin.com or write to PO Box 4797, Hilton Head Island, SC 29938-4797.

Colleen Wracker R.D. is a registered dietitian from Columbia, South Carolina where she works as a nutrition specialist for Richland Memorial Hospital. She has worked in clinical dietetics for ten years specializing in weight management and cardiac rehabilitation programs. The Marian College, Indianapolis graduate is married and lives in Columbia, South Carolina.

From the same author…

10 Steps to a Great Relationship
What every couple should know about love

In his latest book, Dr Howard Rankin, explores the secrets of a great relationship and describes the ten steps that make for real love.

Discover…

- The dynamics of attraction

- The five stages of a relationship

- How to keep romance alive

- Ten rules of fighting fair

- The secrets of intimacy

- How to communicate more effectively

- How to keep your independence in a relationship

- How, when and why to practice forgiveness

- And much more!

$11.95   ISBN# 0-9658261-2-0
Published by Stepwise Press. Distributed by Access Publishers Network.

Available at booksellers or direct by calling 803-842-7797.

From Dr. Howard J. Rankin…

Get Motivated Get Smart Get Slim!

This original tape series includes some of the material of *7 Steps to Wellness* on six audiotapes,. Narrated by the author, the tapes include sections on motivation, self-management, mindfulness, bingeing, temptation management, coping and dealing with others. It also includes motivational link exercises and imagery with realistic sounds which really help to reprogram your key associations.

A bonus tape includes "A Personal Message," designed to help you through the day and keep motivation high.

As well as the 14 day menu plan, the nutrition and exercise guides, the Personal healthscope and Dining-out guide come in handy, wallet-size booklets. There are also motivational stickers to keep you focused on your goals!

Nutritional information and recipes by renowned dietitian Colleen Wracker R.D.

Get Motivated Get Smart Get Slim is available by calling 803-842-7797

We are on the Internet! Visit us at the following locations..

www.relationships_steps.com
Look here for information about *10 Step to a Great Relationship*. The site contains news about updates and other related products as well as seminars, workshops and retreats.

www.wellness_steps.com
This site contains information about the book *7 Steps to Wellness*. It, too, contains information about updates, new products, seminars, workshops and retreats.

www.communication_steps.com
This site contains information about workshops and seminars for professionals. Includes information on the continuing education programs on communication for health-related and other professionals.

www.motivation_steps.com
This site contains information on the *Get Motivated Get Smart Get Slim* program. It also includes information about motivation seminars and workshops.

www.howardrankin.com
This site provides information about Dr. Howard J. Rankin, Howard J. Rankin & Associates Inc., and Stepwise Press Inc., including professional activities and publications.